THE 9-STAR PATIENT EXPERIENCE:
MOMENTS OF MAGIC PLAYBOOK

**For ENCHANTING Your
DENTAL PATIENTS
Into Raving Fans That Pay More,
Refer A Lot More & Stay For A Lifetime**
(even after a pandemic)

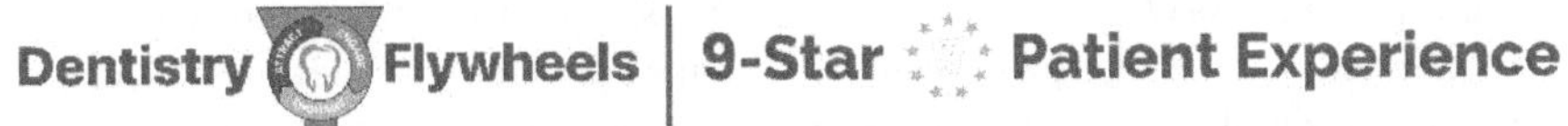

FARAI KUFAKWEDU

Your Practice's Explosive Growth Awaits…

THE 9-STAR
PATIENT EXPERIENCE:

MOMENTS OF MAGIC PLAYBOOK

**For ENCHANTING Your
DENTAL PATIENTS
Into Raving Fans That Pay More,
Refer A Lot More & Stay For A Lifetime**
(even after a pandemic)

Copyright ©   2020 by Farai Kufakwedu

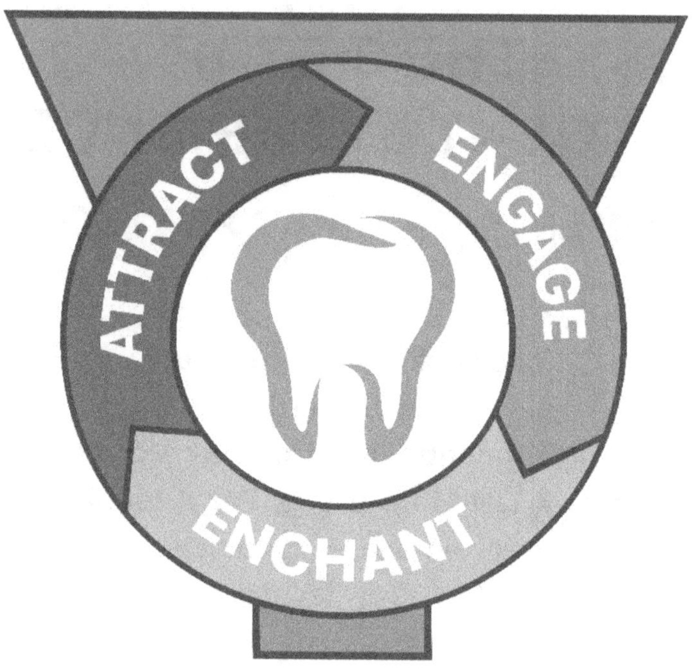

The dentist in your area who will know how to combine
Dentistry Funnels with **Dentistry Flywheels** will
outgrow every other dental practice… guaranteed.

Farai Kufakwedu

To my three kids, Tanyaradzwa,
Ruvimbo and Zvikomborero…
If I've been hard on you, you're welcome.
The world has no patience
for soft people.

TABLE OF CONTENTS

SECTION 0 xiii

THE BACKSTORY xv

WHAT'S A 9-STAR PATIENT EXPERIENCE? xxvii

WHY A 9-STAR PATIENT EXPERIENCE? xxix

THE FIVE ABSOLUTE IMPERATIVES xxxi

SECTION 1 1

MAKE YOUR PATIENTS FEEL CARED FOR

Moment of Magic #1 THE ROYAL THANK YOU 2

Moment of Magic #2 MAKE THE PATIENT FEEL HEARD 4

Moment of Magic #3 MAKE PATIENTS PART OF YOUR TEAM 6

Moment of Magic #4 USE THE POWER OF CELEBRITY 9

Moment of Magic #5 A VALENTINE'S LIKE NO OTHER 11

Moment of Magic #6 THE JOY OF MAKING A DECISION 13

Moment of Magic #7 USE THE BILL CLINTON CHARM 15

Moment of Magic #8 DON'T TALK MONEY LAST 18

Moment of Magic #9 OFFER TO CHARGE THEIR DEVICES 20

Moment of Magic #10 GIVE THE GOLDEN BUSINESS CARD 22

Moment of Magic #11 GIVE THEM THE RED-CARPET TREATMENT 24

Moment of Magic #12 THE DISCOUNTED CAR WASH 27

Moment of Magic #13 THE BIRTHDAY SURPRISE 29

Moment of Magic #14 ASK AFTER THEIR LOVED ONES…BY NAME 31

Moment of Magic #15 HANG THEM ON THE WALL OF FAME 34

Moment of Magic #16 NEVER FUMBLE THEIR NAMES 36

Moment of Magic #17 BRING IN THE PATIENT WITH RESPECT 38

Moment of Magic #18 GIVE THEM A TASTE OF VIP SPA TREATMENTS ...40

SECTION 2 43
YOUR OFFICE'S PERSONALITY

Moment of Magic #19   DITCH THE HOSPITAL SMELL 44

Moment of Magic #20   MAKE THE PATIENT FEEL CALM 46

Moment of Magic #21   SAY NO TO ANXIETY-INSPIRING WALLS 48

Moment of Magic #22   UPGRADE YOUR BEVERAGES............................50

Moment of Magic #23   BREAK BREAD WITH YOUR PATIENTS 52

SECTION 3 55
THE DIGITAL EXPERIENCE

Moment of Magic #24   BE FRIENDLY…ON ALL DEVICES......................57

Moment of Magic #25   DEVELOP A MAGNETIC DIGITAL PERSONA 58

Moment of Magic #26   THE MAGNETIC DIGITAL WELCOME 60

Moment of Magic #27   BE THEIR FAITHFUL GUIDE..............................63

Moment of Magic #28   MAKE THEM ITCH TO GET YOUR OFFERS 66

Moment of Magic #29   MAKE THEM WANT TO KNOW MORE 68

SECTION 4 71
THE COMMUNITY EXPERIENCE

Moment of Magic #30   ENDEAR YOURSELF TO THE COMMUNITY.......72

Moment of Magic #31   SHOW LOVE ON YOUR PATIENTS' CLIENTS..........75

Moment of Magic #32   MAKE IT EASY FOR PEOPLE TO PICK YOU 77

Moment of Magic #33   INVEST IN THE COMMUNITY 79

Moment of Magic #34   BRING THE COMMUNITY TOGETHER 82

Moment of Magic #35   CELEBRATE YOUR PATIENTS 84

Moment of Magic #36   GIFT THEM BOOKS THEY LOVE 86

SECTION 5 89
MAKE THEM FEEL SAFE

Moment of Magic #37   REMOVE MAGNETS FOR VIRUSES.....................90

Moment of Magic #38   BE A CLEAN FREAK 92

Moment of Magic #39   THE CAR WAITING ROOM 94

Moment of Magic #40   NO MORE OPENING DOORS 96

Moment of Magic #41   GIVE AN OFFICE TOUR LIKE NO OTHER..........97

SECTION 6..99

THE 9-STAR FOLLOW UP

Moment of Magic #42 DON'T CARE FOR THEIR MONEY ONLY..........100

Moment of Magic #43 CONTINUE CARING EVEN WHEN THEY STOP...103

Moment of Magic #44 DON'T ANNOY PATIENTS 106

Moment of Magic #45 SURPRISE THEM WITH A POST-OP CALL..........108

SECTION 7..111

THE 9-STAR TEAM EXPERIENCE

Moment of Magic #46 THE 9-STAR TEAM EXPERIENCE 113

Moment of Magic #47 A FUN-FILLED OFFICE DOESN'T SUCK..........114

Moment of Magic #48 A TEAM THAT READS TOGETHER LEADS 116

Moment of Magic #49 USE FBI TYPE INTEL ON YOUR STAFF 118

Moment of Magic #50 LOVE ON YOUR TEAM'S LOVED ONES.............120

Moment of Magic #51 FRESHEN UP YOUR TEAM'S LOOK 122

Moment of Magic #52 BUILD A TEAM OF FBI AGENTS 124

SECTION 8..127

THE 9-STAR PATIENT EXPERIENCE

Moment of Magic #53 DITCH THE PAPER AND CLIP BOARD 128

Moment of Magic #54 MAKE YOUR EQUIPMENT BENEFITS SIZZLE...130

Moment of Magic #55 THE ART OF BUILDING UP THE DENTIST 133

Moment of Magic #56 SOLIDIFY THEIR TRUST IN YOU 135

Moment of Magic #57 SURPRISE THEM WITH A WELCOME CALL......137

SECTION 8..141

CASE ACCEPTANCE EXPLODING EXPERIENCE

Moment of Magic #58 DON'T BREAK THE THREE RINGS RULE..........142

Moment of Magic #59 ASK FOR PERMISSION FIRST..............................145

Moment of Magic #60 USE PHONE EXCITEMENT TO PULL THEM IN...147

Moment of Magic #61 WOW THEM WITH GENUINE INTEREST.......... 151

Moment of Magic #62 DRIVE URGENCY TO HAVE TREATMENT 154

Moment of Magic #63   GIVE THEM ACCESS TO FINER THINGS...........157
Moment of Magic #64   GO VIRTUAL...159
Moment of Magic #65   ASK FOR PERMISSION FIRST............................160

SECTION 9..**161**
THE 9-STAR SOCIAL MEDIA EXPERIENCE
Moment of Magic #66   EXPLODE SAFETY AWARENESS 162
Moment of Magic #67   BE SUPER RESPONSIVE....................................164
Moment of Magic #68   MAKE IT EASY TO LEAVE YOU REVIEWS 166
Moment of Magic #69   LEVERAGE THE POWER OF VIDEO 168
Moment of Magic #70   LOVE ON YOUR PAID LEADS............................170
Moment of Magic #71   TURN UNHAPPY PATIENTS INTO RAVING FANS..172
Moment of Magic #72   APOLOGIZE LIKE NO OTHER 174

CONCLUSION **177**
ACKNOWLEDGEMENTS **179**
ABOUT THE AUTHOR..**181**
ENDNOTES **183**

LIST OF ILLUSTRATIONS

Fig 1: Is Your Practice (Cart) Before Your Horse (Marketing)? xv

Fig 2: Head Concierge's Front Desk Name Plate xxv

Fig 3: Pulling Your Practice On Flat Tires? xxx

Fig 4: Again… What's Pulling What? xxxii

Fig 5: The 5 Absolute Imperatives xxxiii

Fig 6: Gain An Unfair Advantage 5

Fig 7: Survey Text Message 8

Fig 8: Story Of Two New Patient Pipelines 10

Fig 9: Holes In Your Practice Balloon? 17

Fig 9: Are You Flushing Money Down The Toilet? 21

Fig 10: Focusing On The Wrong Things? 30

Fig 11: Viral Patient Experience 47

Fig 12: Are You Shooting Yourself In The Foot? 49

Fig 13: Is Your Digital Presence Sleeping On the Job? 56

Fig 14: Is Your Web Copy Narcissistic? 62

Fig 15: The Dentistry Funnel 65

Fig 16: Treatment Page Sample 70

Fig 17: Shooting Yourself In The Foot? 74

Fig 18: Nelson Ridge Dental Giving Back 81

Fig 19: Demonstrating You Care…Like Friend 102

Fig 20: Patient Reactivation Postcard Sample 104

Fig 21: Patient Reactivation Text Message 105

Fig 22: Marketing Automation Dashboard 107

Fig 23: Sample Dentist Follow Up Text 109

Fig 24: Focusing On The Wrong Things? 112

Fig 25: Go Digital With Patient Information Collection 129

Fig 26: Burning Cash Through Advertising? 132

Fig 27: Dentist's New Patient WOW Text 139

Fig 28: Dr. Money Bags vs Dr. Pickup Scraps 144

Fig 29: Excitement Must Show Through The Phone 150

Fig 30: Crush Your Competition 156

Fig 31: Respond To Social Media Reviews 165

Fig 32: Reviews Request Email 167

Fig 33: Reviews Notification Text 173

SECTION 0

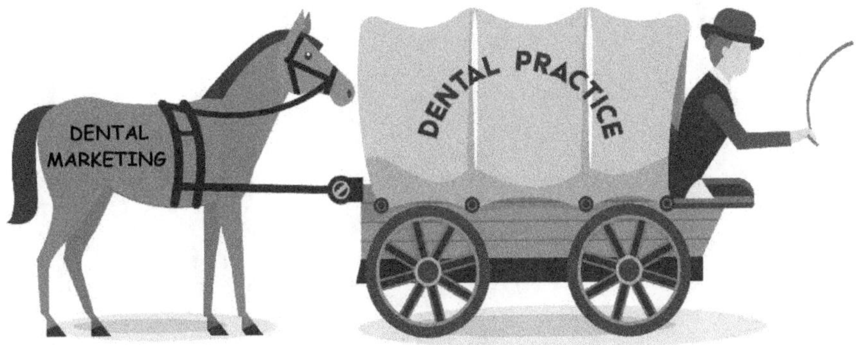

**Fig 1: Is Your Practice (Cart)
Before Your Horse (Marketing)?**

The smart dentist does not build a practice without
understanding how he or she is in the business of
marketing his or her dental practice. That's like putting
the horse before the cart. It just doesn't work.

Farai Kufakwedu

THE BACKSTORY

TORTURED AND HUNGRY... IMMIGRANT FINDS GOLD LINING THE STREETS OF TORONTO

I came to Canada from Zimbabwe in 2001 with fresh torture wounds still oozing blood on my back - literally. I had to change shirts several times during the 13-hour flight from Johannesburg to Toronto because the shirts kept sticking onto my wounds as I sat on the plane. I was running for my life, but I was also hungry for opportunity and man oh man, did the first world come through? You bet it did.

As an African young man who had never been to the developed world, living in a metropolitan city in North America shocked my system like nothing had ever done before. It took me a while to figure things out, but figure them I did eventually. As I settled into life in the city in the coming next few years, I finally came to find gold in the form of business opportunities literally lining the streets of the mega city.

THE BIG DREAMS OF AN ENTREPRENEURIAL SPIRITED IMMIGRANT

Fast forward to 2011. I was now a father of two beautiful girls, Mary-Angel and Victoria. I had been in Canada for a decade. Having had a business of one kind or another during my university years in Zimbabwe, when I escaped to Canada, never was there a time when I was under the illusion that true freedom in life would be achieved while working for somebody else. Having grown up poor, the only avenue to freedom I knew was by building a business. All the people I knew that were rich – not counting corrupt politicians – were businessmen. So, starting a business was top of my mind even when I was changing my bloodied shirts during the two legs of my dreadfully long flight to Canada.

So in 2011, I was two years into building and running my first business - GreenWill Concierge & Security Services. Having worked as a security guard during all my years studying Chemical Engineering at Ryerson University in Toronto, and being armed with a Marketing Degree from N.U.S.T in Zimbabwe, I was confident of my ability to offer much better security and concierge services to condominium residents and the property management companies that ran them.

COMING FACE TO FACE WITH THE MIGHTY WALL

By 2011, my company had 9 contracts, about 25 employees and doing about $30,000 in gross revenue per month. My company was offering generic front desk, concierge, and physical security services. Nothing special. My client base was made up of middle income high-rise residential condominiums. From the way I saw things, we were struggling to grow. The profit margins in commoditized physical security are slim. Very slim.

My staff turnover was off the wall because I paid the bare minimum. I paid the bare minimum because my clients paid the bare minimum. Two years into starting the company, my future was not looking as bright as I thought it would be. Competition was as stiff as the manhood of a dude who's just met his wife for the first time after five years in prison. I was constantly tired, not to mention the fact that I had my phone on all the time, including bedtime. If something went wrong, like a major incident happening at one of our buildings, I had to go. And we had a lot of major incidents.

Being clueless and hungry for success, I figured that if I get a lot more clients, my problems would somehow solve themselves. My beast mode was turned on every day. I see many dentists doing the same thing with their maniacal focus on getting new patients. So, I was hitting the streets of Toronto hard, going building to building talking to condominium managers, asking if their buildings' physical security and concierge services contracts were coming up for renewal.

My prospecting strategy was very simple. I'd drive to a high-rise building, park my car in the visitor parking lot and go straight into the building's lobby. I'd take a few minutes to survey the front desk operation. I'd take note of the concierge/security company serving the building, how many people were staffing the front desk and observe the resident traffic in and out of the building. I'd then ask to see the property manager, who in most cases, would be happy to see me.

When I got into the property manager's office, I'd introduce myself, make small talk to build rapport based on what I observed in the lobby and front desk. I'd then ask the property manager when their security and concierge services contract would be up for renewal. I'd also ask if they would let us present a proposal when that time comes. In most cases, the property manager would agree, and I'd come out knowing when a contract was coming up, which security company was in place and which management company was running the building. I'd do my prospecting rounds for three to five hours daily depending on what else was going on in the business.

Once I had completed the section of the city that I had planned to prospect in, I would get into my car and drive to my office to continue the day. To say building the business was tough would be to understate things. I would be as tired as hell and would be feeling the way an ultra-marathon runner feels at the end of day one in a three-day race knowing fully the same pain is coming tomorrow. I loved building my business, just as much as you love building your dental practice; don't get me wrong. And believe it or not, I loved my clients…most of the time, but I was facing a mighty wall that I didn't know how to go over. I wanted to grow but I was afraid that growth would bring me more of the same clients that I have. This would only multiply my problems. And the profits with those types of clients wouldn't be any better. Something had to give. I just had no [expletive] clue what.

THE DAY EVERYTHING CHANGED

One afternoon as I was doing my regular prospecting rounds, the lobby door to a building I was about to enter was opened for me by a smartly dressed gentleman in white gloves. This had never happened before. Of all the buildings I had been into – and believe me when I say I had been into hundreds of buildings - none had a person whose role was to open the door for residents and visitors to come in or go out. I was warmly greeted and directed to the front desk where a male and female were working behind a large lobby counter serving people. As I looked around to familiarize myself, I immediately felt that I was in a different world. A completely different world from anything that I had experienced before in real life.

Do you remember the scene in Black Panther when Everest Ross woke up in Shuri's lab in Wakanda? Do you remember how shockingly surprised Ross looked and felt? (If you want to refresh your memory, just do a quick search on YouTube. Type Everest Ross

Wakes up in Wakanda.) That…is exactly how I felt and looked as I took in this new world I had just stumbled into.

See… I grew up in Dzivaresekwa, one of the poorest high-density suburbs in Zimbabwe's capital, Harare. I'd never in my entire life entered a place such as this. The personality of the building was that of luxury. I could smell, see, hear, and feel an aura that screamed; RICH PEOPLE LIVE HERE!! And indeed, they did. The paintings on the walls, the lobby furnishings, the color themes and lastly, the people walking in, out and around, all whispered sophistication and wealth. I was blown away. As I was taking in this blissful experience, I was awakened from my reverie by a very gentle, but lively voice.

"Good afternoon Sir, you seem to have been taken in by the place. I saw you come in after Dave opened the door, but I didn't want to disturb you, seeing how engrossed and pleasurably fascinated you're taking in our place. How may I be of assistance today?"

My experience just got blown into space at that point. If I thought this was a well-run place from just looking and experiencing the ambiance and personality of the lobby, I was just about to get my socks blown off by the quality of service offered by the front desk and concierge staff.

Ron, the guy who I was talking to, I came to learn, was the Valet, and wanted to know if I needed to have my car parked if I was staying for more than 30 minutes.

Holy Christ almighty!!! What place is this? I thought to myself. They even park your car for you? Jesus Christ!! And the uniform those people were wearing?!! Oh my God!! The level of service those front desk people were delivering as I watched them interact with visitors and residents just about blew my brains out. I think my mouth was wide open all the time and I must have whispered the phrase Holy

Sh** under my breath enough times to put a nun into a coma. I was blown away.

It was in this moment that I realized there was no way the company these people worked for could lose this contract. Their service was just too good to replace.

After a good 20 or so minutes talking to the staff, I went in to speak to the Property Manager who continued the journey of service I had had the first taste of the moment I walked into the building. When I asked him when his current concierge contract would be up for renewal, he told me point blank that Forest Hill Valet (now the Forest Hill Group) will never be replaced. Not unless the company gets out of business, or if something crazy like that happens. According to him, his condo board members would have him fired were he to just as much as mention the idea of replacing the current company and its staff. That's how good their service was.

A NEW PLAN IS BORN

When I left the building, I didn't continue prospecting. I couldn't continue. I just couldn't. My head was spinning way too fast, but I could see clearly now. It's like a colored layer of glasses had been taken off my direction of sight and I could see the world in a new way. Like Dabasir in George S. Clason's *Richest Man in Babylon*; "All the world seemed to be of a different color as though I had been looking at it through a colored stone which had suddenly been removed… With a new vision, I saw the things that I must do."[1]

Even though it was now late afternoon, I didn't go home. I drove straight to my office. I called my young brother who worked with me to go around the properties we looked after to make sure everything was fine and then to take the rest of the day off. I told him I just met God and I was going to the office to write down what he told me concerning GreenWill, our business. I called my wife and gave her the long and short of my just ended encounter with God. I informed her that I would not be coming home until I have completed putting down on paper what was on my mind. And believe when I say this… there was a lot on my mind.

As I made my way to the office on Toronto's Highway 401, my mind became fully made up on the course of action needed to not only take GreenWill to the next level but also on the course of action needed to get my family and I the freedom I've have always dreamed of. To build the company and life of my dreams, this is what I was going to do.

I was going to change my service offering by exponentially upgrading it to focus 100% on providing the highest level of customer service possible and then targeting high-end properties in my prospecting. I was going to change my uniform to a very upscale look and I was going to study how things are done at any upscale hotel or residential building I could find in the city. I was going to put on both my student engineering and marketing hats and study-up heavy on the business of serving rich people living in high-rise buildings. But more than anything else, I was going to implement whatever I learnt. Even while I was serving middle-income residents whose boards were paying me peanuts.

PERSISTING THROUGH THE GROWING PAINS

In the weeks that followed, I had one-on-one meetings with each and every one of my employees during their days off. I would visit them in their neighborhoods, and we'd go for coffee to talk. I got to put together a comprehensive set of procedures on every possible touchpoint between my staff and the residents we would be serving. I looked up experts in training and had my staff receive the training they needed to deliver the level of service expected in the upscale buildings, even while we were still serving only middle-class income residents.

One of the biggest push backs I got right away was from the staff complaining that they were not paid enough to give the level of service I was asking them to give. Which was a fair point. So I increased the wages to the point of not being able to make our own financial obligations as a family. I paid my staff to go and observe how things were done at upscale hotels in the city. I contracted one of Toronto's most prominent majordomos (*the head servant who acts on behalf of the owner of a large or significant residence*). to provide training to my team knowing that when it comes to making rich people happy, nothing would be off limits as long as it was within the bounds of the law.

Getting all my teams across the city to adopt the same mindset, get on board my vision and have everyone working from the same script was hard. But I was determined. The image of people in my uniforms working in high-end buildings, serving high-class residences had branded itself into my mind. There was no way getting rid of it except by making it a reality.

NOTHING TASTES SWEETER THAN VICTORY

Fast forward a year and half later. We had grown from around 30 people to 100 full-time staff. We were averaging about $150,000 in gross revenue per month and more upscale clients were knocking on our doors. Gone were the days of hitting the pavements knocking on property managers' doors. GreenWill Security & Concierge Services had become one of a handful of companies in Toronto providing bespoke security and front desk, concierge, and valet services to the highly price insensitive residents who lived in some of Toronto's upscale high-rise buildings.

Just take a look at the glass name plates below that our Head Concierge put on the lobby counter to welcome residents and visitors. This just goes to show you that indeed, we were playing the upscale service game on another level.

Fig 2: Head Concierge's Front Desk Name Plate

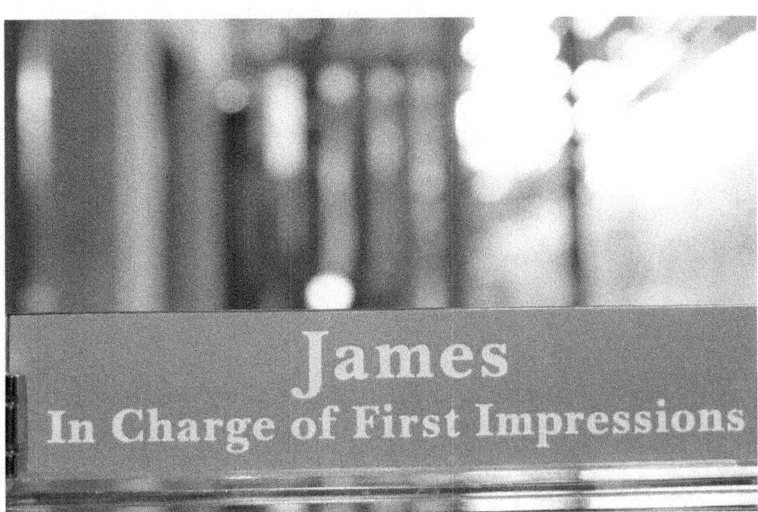

We were able to secure contracts that allowed us to pay our staff wages and benefits that were way above industry averages. This made our turnover drop like an iron ball. High quality people were knocking on our door looking for work. I was able to bring in people with leadership skills to run the day to day operations at our buildings which freed my time to focus on my girls. Because of the high-profile nature of some of our buildings, I was approached by a bigger company looking to buy me out and I took the best offer to exit the business.

WHAT ALL THIS HAS TO DO WITH YOU…

By now you must be wondering what all this has to do with you. You are a dental practice owner, why am I talking about how my unknown company grew 5X in the short space of 1.5 years by focusing on delivering an outstanding, white glove customer experience for our residents?

Well, I'm telling you about this because you are not an ordinary dental practice owner. If you were, you'd not be reading the playbook on moments of magic to help you deliver a 9-star patient experience. You're a dentist who understands the following critical fact - the same fact that Horst Schulze understood when he co-founded the Ritz-Carlton Hotel group. You understand this same fact that everybody you know who has built a wildly successful dental practice understands and it is this…

Delivering a world-class patient experience is the only key to building a great business.

Delivering a world-class experience for your patients is what this book is about. To borrow a fine concept from Horst Schulze,[2] your patients want three main things.

Thing #1: They want dental services with no defects.
Thing #2: They want timeliness.
Thing #3: They want you and your team to be nice to them.

This book is about getting Thing #3 done very well. Why? Because it is excelling on Thing #3 that will ensure your practice grows to give you the life that you want for yourself, your loved ones and for everyone whose life and happiness depends on the success of your practice.

THE GOAL OF THIS BOOK

My singular goal with this book is to provide you, the savvy dental practice owner and your leadership team, with strategies you can execute on to deliver a patient experience that will get people to pay you for more treatment, stay with you longer and for them to refer a lot more of their friends and loved ones to your practice.

You will, therefore, find that apart from this section of the book, everything else is practical strategy that must be executed on. If you are a man or a woman who values action over talk, and you have your sights set on building one of the most remarkable dental practices in the country, then this book is a must read for you and everybody on your team.

Ok, now that we have dispensed with the introductions, like my man Jocko Willink likes to say…let's get it done.

WHAT'S A 9-STAR PATIENT EXPERIENCE?

Before we get into the meat and potatoes of the strategies in the book, I think it's a good idea for us to be on the same page regarding what exactly is meant by **The 9-Star Patient Experience.**

Consider the customer service experience you would enjoy if you were a guest at a Ritz-Carlton or the Four Seasons hotel. Or consider the customer service experience a person gets if they are a first-class passenger aboard an Emirates flight. That is 5-Star service. Anybody who goes through this experience the first time will always come back for more if they could afford it.

Now imagine if that uber high-end customer service experience were to be upgraded four notches higher so that instead of the 5-Star service, it becomes a 9-Star service or a 9-Star Experience. That, I'm sure you'd agree, would be an experience out of this world. One that anybody who gets it for the first time would come back for more and tell all their loved ones, hated ones (through social media posts), friends, and enemies.

That over the top customer service experience is what this book is all about. It is about delivering a dental experience so out of this world your patients will love you so much that they will come back for more treatment, stay with you forever and create a flood of referrals into your practice.

Now… in order to deliver the 9-Star Experience, you're going to need delivery vehicles. Your delivery vehicles are the many possible touchpoints between the patients and your team. Let's borrow a term from the great Dr. David Moffet[3] and call these touch points Moments of Magic. It is the cumulative effect of all the Moments of Magic that will make up the patients' 9-Star Experience with your practice.

To define the 9-Star Patient Experience using an adaptation of Dan Kennedy's Engineering The Practice For Environmental Effectives; the 9-Star Patient Experience is… "one that in every way makes the patient feel welcome, respected, appreciated and valued, builds understanding and compliance through education, creates and strengthens trust, and stimulates direct referrals as well as word of mouth advertising"

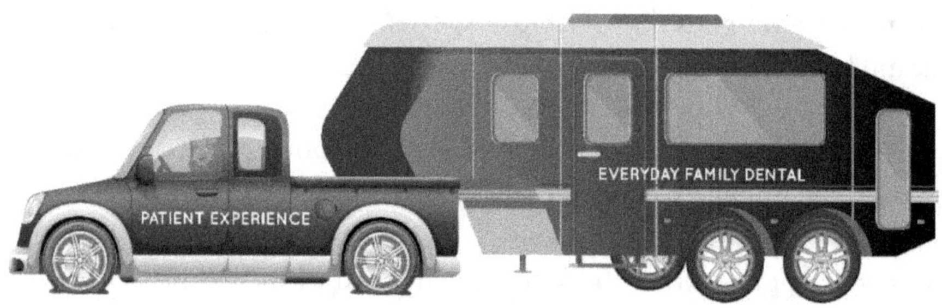

Fig 3: Pulling Your Practice On Flat Tires?

The patient experience is the truck that will pull your dental practice 'camper'. If that truck's wheels are flat; well, you know how far you will go with your desire to work less and build the practice of your dreams. You won't go far. Believe it!

WHY THE FOCUS ON DELIVERING A 9-STAR PATIENT EXPERIENCE?

According to a RightNow Technologies Customer Experience Report, 86% of U.S. adults are willing to pay more for a better customer experience and 73% of U.S. adults said they fell in love with a brand as a result of the brand's customer service. Today's patients don't just want generic products and services, they want, and have come to expect unique experiences that they can't get anywhere else.[4]

The savvy dental practice owner, therefore, thrives because he or she understands and takes action on the fact that his or her patients would pay for more treatment, be loyal, and would refer a lot more of their friends and loved ones if they are delighted with the experience they are given.

At a time when 68% of customers say they'd leave a service provider because they believe the business does not care about them, the smart dentist goes an extra nine miles to put in place people and systems that remove any signs of indifference in his or her team.

With the ever-increasing threat of deep-pocketed DSOs breathing on the necks of independent private practices, the savvy dentist takes a leaf out of Dr. Paul Etchison's playbook to "create such a great patient experience that people will be willing to accept the lack of convenience as a tradeoff for the outstanding care that they receive."

Fig 4: Again... What's Pulling What?

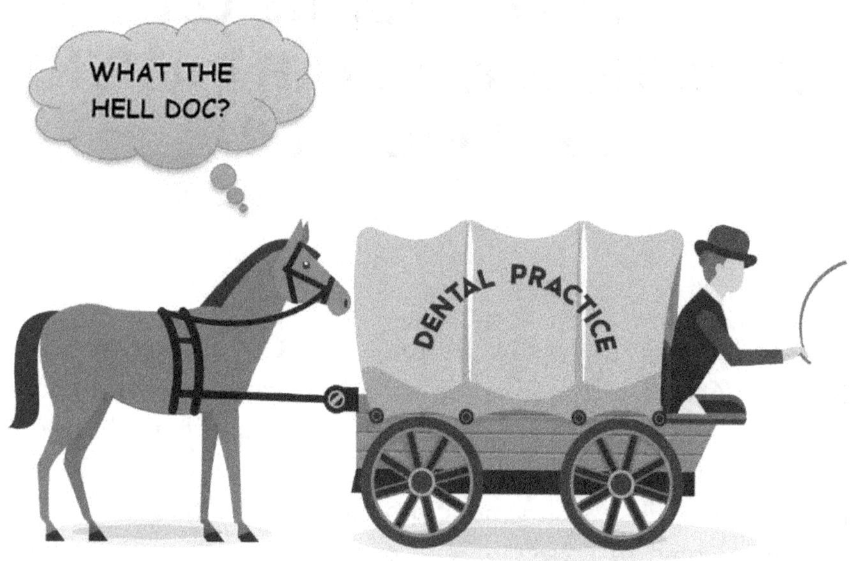

If the patient experience were the horse and your dental practice the cart, it's not your practice's growth that will determine the patient experience. It is the current and prospective patients' experience with your practice that determines the growth and impact your practice will have on you, your family, and your team. The dentist who understands this universal truth will retire sooner, richer, and having made a far greater impact in the lives of his patients and his team.

The dentist who understands this and takes no action and the dentist who doesn't understand this will be forced to work till they grow old, will make very insignificant impact on their community, family and team, and will be forced to sell their practices for cents on the dollar when they're finally forced to retire. You have a choice to make. Get in touch and let's work together.

THE FIVE ABSOLUTE IMPERATIVES

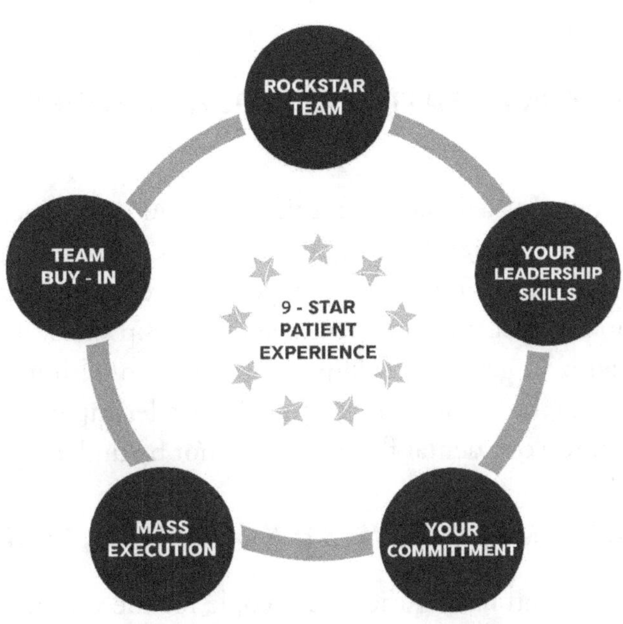

Fig 5: The 5 Absolute Imperatives

For your practice to succeed in delivering the 9-Star Patient Experience, five things must be present. These are the Five Absolute Imperatives without which it is impossible to build a practice that will guarantee your financial future. If you miss one of the absolute imperatives, it doesn't matter how well you do in the execution of the other four, your dental business will struggle. If you miss two or more, then your practice has no chance of thriving in the unforgiving post Covid-19 economy.

ABSOLUTE IMPERATIVE #1: YOUR COMMITMENT

When asked what separates the top 10% of dentists from the bottom 90%, Dr. Justin Short - co-author of the book, Titans of Dentistry, and the driver behind The Lifestyle Practice - said it was <u>proper mindset</u> and the <u>willingness to work hard</u> that separate the 90% strugglers from the thriving 10%5. You have to be committed to working hard in executing these strategies in order to realize their benefits.

ABSOLUTE IMPERATIVE #2: YOUR LEADERSHIP SKILLS

Like John Maxell said, everything falls and rises on leadership.[6] To grow your practice into becoming a place where patients are excited to come to is going to require you to excel as a leader. Because growing an elite practice requires great leadership skills, if you don't have one already, get a leadership mentor and go all in towards the execution of his or her advice. The role that leadership plays in giving momentum to your dental flywheel must not be understated.

ABSOLUTE IMPERATIVE #3: YOUR ROCKSTAR TEAM

Selecting and having the right people for the various functions in your practice is an absolute must. Your drive to deliver a 9-Star Patient Experience starts with your team or else it doesn't have a chance at all. When I grew my concierge and valet services business from $30,000 monthly revenues to $150,000 in the short space of one and half years, it was only because I went to heaven and back to bring in the right people for the various roles I needed played.

Likewise, if you are going to give your patients a 9-Star Experience, you have to do whatever it takes to select and bring in people with the right attitudes and personalities. After you have found these awesome people and brought them in, you need to get their buy in because without it, it won't matter how good they are.

ABSOLUTE IMPERATIVE #4: TEAM BUY-IN

Nothing of permanent value is going to happen without 100% buy-in from your internal customers - your team. Delivering intensely patient-centric service is not possible without having the absolute buy-in of the people responsible for the delivery of that service experience. Having your entire team to fully understand that it's their future and that of their loved ones that's at stake will go a long way in getting that buy in. There are many books, podcast episodes, and training programs on the market to help you build the team you need.

ABSOLUTE IMPERATIVE #5: MASSIVE EXECUTION

Taking massive action in the deployment of the strategies outlined in this book is what will ultimately separate the dentists that will have multiple six, seven, and eight figure dental practices from those that will be barely struggling to get by. Now, it's important to take note of the following important fact...

You don't have to try and implement all the strategies at the same time. It's impossible. You pick the strategies you can deploy right away and go from there. The key is to start taking action.

SECTION 1

MAKE YOUR PATIENTS FEEL CARED FOR

THE ROYAL THANK YOU

GIVE PATIENTS WHO REFER A 'THANK YOU' LIKE NO OTHER

Fred Joyal, the legendary dentistry marketing strategist, is big on creating experiences that reward patients for sending referrals. According to Fred, getting an active referrals generation machine firing on all cylinders requires a well-thought-out rewards program.

How much is a patient worth to your practice over the course of their life? How much is the same patient worth to you, your family, and your staff when you consider the referrals they send your way? A whole lot! So, what do you think would make Linda feel special and appreciated after she has referred a mom with a family of 3 teens to your practice? What would make Linda swear her dentist's office is the best thing since sliced bread after she has done you a solid by sending a high value referral?[7]

Depending on the week (always theme your weeks based on public holidays, anniversaries, or other special days) when the referral comes in, you can create a library of experiences that wow your patients.

Let's suppose Loice and her family (the referred) had their referral appointment during Linda's (the referrer) birthday week. Now in order to create the most awesome referral reward experience for Linda, you must consider the fact that she has, at zero cost to you, referred a family of 5 into your practice. Now, let me take my family of 5 for example.

In 2019 we represented about $17,000 worth of dental benefits based on our benefits plan. Now suppose we qualified for, or were in need of just $10,000 worth of dental care, not the entire $17,000. If we stay at our dentist for 10 years before we leave the city, that is a whopping $100,000 worth of collections that a dental practice would get from us referred patients.

So, what would a one time thank you experience look like for somebody who just brought you $100,000 worth of business? I'll let you decide what you believe is appropriate, but I'll say this; Linda will be calling Loice to thank her for taking the advice to choose you as her dentist. Whatever gift you give to Linda, she will be talking about it to all her friends over the phone and on social media.

Now ask yourself this…are you using your referrals rewards as opportunities to create experiences for your patients that make them come back and refer more people? What is the ideal experience you want your clients to have after they send you a referral? If a referred patient is still with you after say, five years, how about surprising the patient who made that referral with some extravagant present or experience?

MAKE THE PATIENT FEEL HEARD

When I was running my concierge, valet, and security business serving upscale condos in Toronto, one of the biggest frustrations for residents was when they felt they were not heard. This happened when they voiced displeasure regarding something they expected to have been handled after they had relayed prior instructions. The feeling of being heard or unheard ranks among the top in determining the experience one has with any service. This is why 68% of people say they will leave a business if they see the business as indifferent.

The potential for making customers feel unheard exponentially rises in situations where an instruction or some information has to be relayed across multiple people. Like in a dental office. When a patient has to repeat his or her concerns multiple times, the feeling of being unheard creeps up several rungs up on the bad experience ladder. You take a page out of Dr. Gina Dorfman's playbook.

According to Dr. Dorfman, the creator of dental software, YAPI, the best way to make patients feel heard is to have your team on the same page 100% of the time. And the best way known to dentistry to get a team start the day on the same page is to prepare for patients in advance during the morning huddle.[8]

This is the perfect time for all members of your team to get themselves acquainted with any concerns patients might have shared. It is also the perfect time to go over any information the patient might have shared that the team can use to create that '*oh-they-remember-this-about-me*' feeling that is so important for creating the awesome experience you want your patients to have.

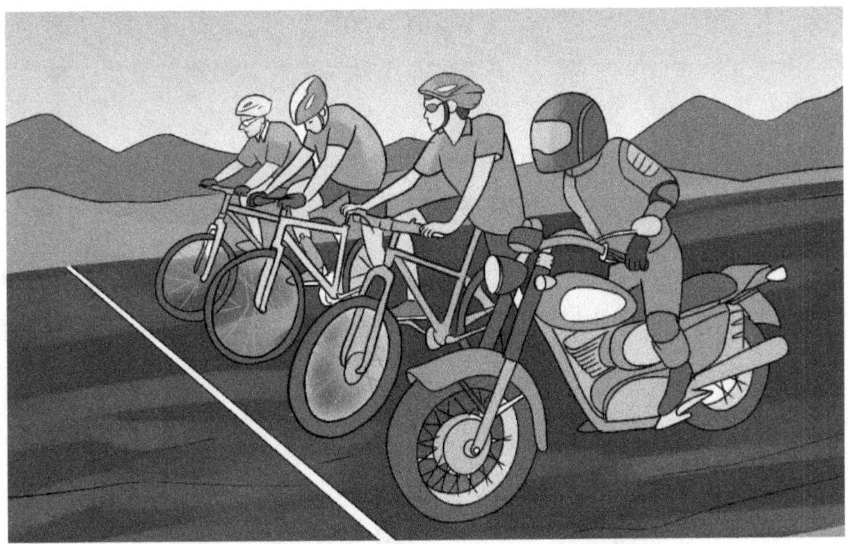

Fig 6: Gain An Unfair Advantage

When compared to the competition, the savvy dentist who makes his or her patients feel heard and cared for has the unfair advantage of a bike racer who competes with other racers riding bicycles. **Which of these four racers would you have your dental practice be?**

MAKE PATIENTS PART OF YOUR TEAM

MAKE YOUR PATIENTS FEEL THEY ARE PART OF SERVICE DELIVERY PROCESS

One of the simplest, yet most important innovations that led to the Ritz-Carlton hotels becoming a world leader in delivering outrageous levels of customer service was the Comments Card System. Comment cards were given to guests so they would have a place to write their comments, suggestions, gripes, and rants.

Horst Schulze and his team realized that people like it when they are made to feel important in a genuine way. People like to be given the opportunity to contribute to something greater than themselves. When Horst asked his guests to join him and his team in identifying areas that needed improvement as the Ritz-Carlton hotels sought to become the most service experience-oriented hotel in the world, people took him up on the offer. The results have been nothing short of amazing in the number of guest comment cards that people have written.

So, like the famed story of the Ritz-Carlton hotels, give your patients the experience of being part of something grand. You're establishing yourself as the center of all things great in the world of top-of-the-class dental experiences in your city; ask your patients to help you deliver on that. Have them give you input and watch. You'll only be disappointed by your failure or inability to execute on some of the great ideas you will get.

But when you implement some of the ideas and communicate that to your community, do you think their bond with your practice will become stronger? Do you think people will personally feel bad if they have to cancel an appointment? You bet they will. Because now they feel they are part of your practice having contributed great ideas on how best to make them happy.

So, create both a physical comments card system and a digital one using patient surveys. Ever since I came to Canada 20 years ago, I am still to be asked for a comment by any one of the dentists I've patronized. The field is therefore wide open for the business savvy dentist who wants to blow everybody out of the water and be the only game in town worth going to.

Fig 7: Survey Text Message

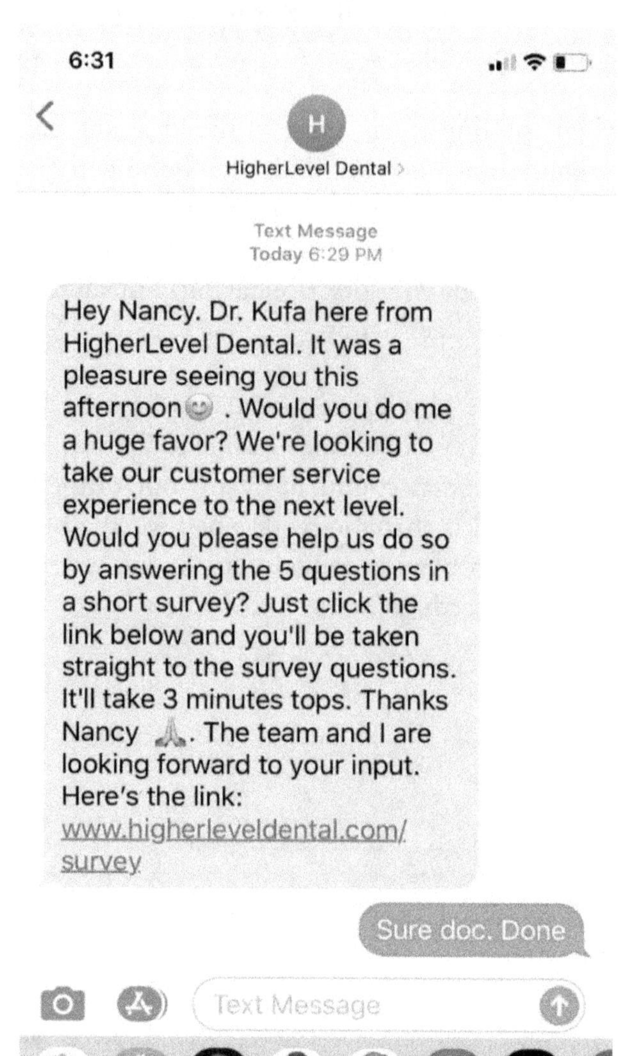

USE THE POWER OF CELEBRITY

MAKE YOUR PATIENTS FEEL GREAT KNOWING THAT SOME IMPORTANT OR FAMOUS PEOPLE ARE PATIENTS OF YOURS

Do you have a celebrity as a patient? Or a sports figure or somebody who is important in some way who is a patient of yours? Say a city councilor or owner of a company? You can use this information to make your patients feel great about having you as their Dentist and bring up the perceived value of your practice.

Why do you think a real estate agent selling a home in a neighborhood where a movie star or pro sports player lives will mention this fact to all prospective home buyers? Because for the buyer, it feels great to tell one's friends that I just bought a house close to such and such celebrity. It's vain I know, but that's how most of the humans you serve are wired. We feel great when we find a way to associate ourselves with the people that society considers successful.

It sure feels great for a patient to know that there is a huge possibility the chair she's sitting in to get her teeth cleaned is the same chair a big celebrity sat in the last he was in here. I mean, who wouldn't want to tell their friends they go to Spodak Dental, the same dental office that Tony Robins goes to?

And… you don't have to violate any privacy laws by giving out the names of the power people who patronize you. Just hinting at the fact alone without divulging any names will do the trick. You can convey this information in a variety of ways. On your website, in your Patient Newsletter, via email or just as part of everyday conversations between your team members and the patients they serve.

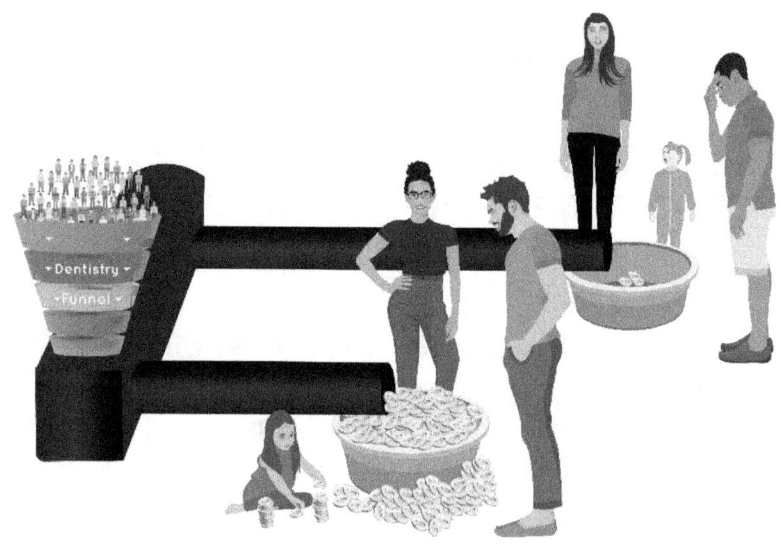

Fig 8: Story Of Two New Patient Pipelines

Appreciating your patients and going out of your way to make sure they know you appreciate them will pay you and your family in ways most dentists will never enjoy. Less stress, more free time to invest in other pursuits that bring you joy and happiness. **Which of these two dental practice owners would your family rather be?**

A VALENTINE'S LIKE NO OTHER

BE THE HIGHLIGHT OF A PATIENT'S VALENTINE'S WEEK

Valentine's Day is one great opportunity to make your patients feel special. The actual strategies deployed are only limited by your team's imaginations and what information you have on your patients.

Use your marketing automation system to segment your patients based on what treatments they have received. You can then design and deploy your Valentine's Week campaigns targeted to individual patients based on the treatments they received. Imagine a patient receiving several personalized messages – a physical Happy Valentine's Card, text message, email, and voice mail – during Valentine's Week. How would this experience make the patient feel?

If you were the patient getting so much positive attention, how would that make you feel? Would you talk about the experience on social media? Would you feel valued and thought of? People love to be validated and acknowledged. A well thought out Valentine's Week strategy would go a long way in solidifying the relationship you have with your patient community.

You can take this strategy to the next level by sending flowers to a select group of patients who have, for instance, brought in a certain number of referrals.

THE JOY OF MAKING A DECISION

HOW GIVING YOUR PATIENTS THE EXPERIENCE OF MAKING AN IMPORTANT DECISION AND TAKING ACTION ON IT WILL TRIPLE YOUR CASE ACCEPTANCE

Humans… we are wired to seek to thrive and when we do, we keep reaching to be more. The pursuit of getting better, becoming more, or achieving more is at the core of what makes us human. It therefore comes as no surprise that people will reward you in proportion to the opportunities you give them to get ahead.

A dentist, more than anybody else, understands that a person's smile - especially in this day and age - is a critical determinant of how far one progresses in life. And people know this. So, when you give a patient the experience of making a decision on a dental treatment you are presenting, you have helped that patient take action on something that is fundamental to them getting ahead in life.

You know how gratifying it is to check off an important task or project as being done at the end of the day. Imagine how grateful your client Debbie feels when she knows you've enabled her to decide on the best teeth alignment option for her daughter Claire. Think about how good she feels as she leaves your office with a decided option as the next step in her daughter's treatment plan. In her mind and in reality, she is thriving and progressing in life…all thanks to you.

So, how do you give your patients the experience of progressing and getting ahead in life? Simple. You take a page out of Dr. Burleson's playbook.

According to Dr. Burleson, the patient will leave your practice enjoying the experience of having chosen a treatment plan's next step only if you and your team don't let them leave with multiple treatment options. By making it a policy that the patient can never leave your office without having decided on ONE treatment option, you give that patient the opportunity to make progress on a very important decision. [9]

Getting a patient to say YES starts with the first treatment case acceptance domino going down. And that domino is having a patient pick one treatment option before they leave the consultation room. Decisions that involve significant financial commitments are difficult to make when there are several options facing us. We always experience feelings of gratefulness for the person who makes it easy for us to choose an option and take the next steps.

So, ask yourself this…are patients leaving your practice with a treatment option having been decided, and clear next steps agreed on or are you letting patients leave your office with several treatment options for them to think over or discuss with their spouses? The former gives your patients the feelings of getting ahead in life, and they will reward you with getting the treatment done while the later will leave your patients with the confusion that comes from indecision, and they will reward you with not taking the action you want.

USE THE BILL CLINTON CHARM

DEPLOY THE BILL CLINTON CHARM TO YOUR PATIENTS AND THEY'LL BELIEVE THERE IS NONE BETTER THAN YOU...AT ANYTHING

I once read somewhere that one of the personality traits that drew people to former President Bill Clinton was his ability to make people - during face-to-face interactions - feel they matter more than anything else the President cared for. Imagine having the experience of feeling you matter more than anything else in the eyes of the President. It is said President Clinton's ability to make regular people feel important was responsible for his major successes as a President.

Now, what does President Clinton's prowess in making people feel important have to do with you delivering a 9-Star Patient Experience as a dentist? Well, this has a lot to do with you because the experience of feeling valued sits at the heart of the remarkable experience your patients crave for.

Have you ever heard the joke of the dentist and his assistant who were discussing their weekend plans while the good doctor worked on one Mr. Jones? Imagine what was going through Mr. Jones' mind as the dentist and his assistant totally ignored the fact that he was fully present and there they were, talking away about their weekend plans as if he wasn't there.

Now, in order for Mr. Jones to have a great treatment experience, he must be made to feel like he is the center of the universe while he sits in your chair. He must be made to feel that way because, indeed, he is the center of the universe as long as your success depends on Mr. Jones' patronage.

So, what do you have to do in order to make Mr. Jones feel the way he is supposed to feel? What needs to happen for your patients to know and feel that they matter while they receive treatment?

According to Dr. David Moffet, there must be zero chit chat between you and your assistant while a patient is being worked on.[10] There must be good-natured, goal-oriented conversation between you and Mr. Jones. Your conduct must demonstrate confidence in your clinical skills while your light conversation continues to create trust building rapport. This is the kind of chairside experience that will keep Mr. Jones paying, staying, and referring more high-quality people your way.

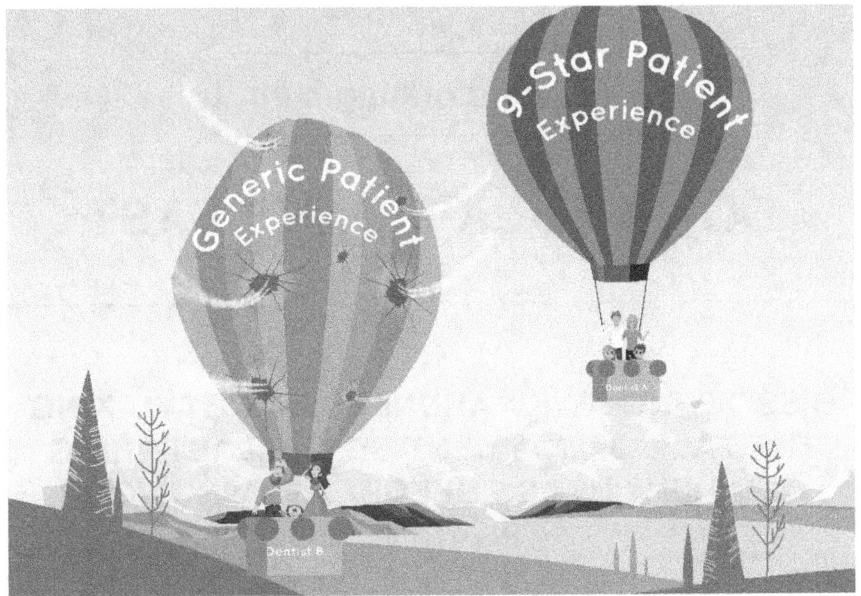

Fig 9: Holes In Your Practice Balloon?

Having your practice be known for giving patients a world-class experience as they interact with your brand digitally or in person can be likened to flying the blue air balloon. It will take you wherever you, your family, and your team wants to go. A practice that does not focus on having a great patient experience, on the other hand, is like flying in the red balloon. What ever your destination is…working less hours, retiring early, selling your practice at a high valuation, less stress, making a bigger impact or whatever, with a balloon riddled with holes, you will not be going anywhere fast. It's time to patch up those holes. Get in touch today. Let's talk strategy. www.9spe.com/contact

DON'T TALK MONEY LAST

DISSOLVING AWKWARDNESS BY NOT MAKING THE TALK OF PAYMENT BE THE LAST THING A PATIENT HEARS BEFORE LEAVING YOUR PRACTICE

The human psyche is by evolution wired to avoid and dislike the loss of one's possessions. Even if the loss of those possessions is due to fair, and sometimes, much needed exchange for other people's services and goods.

People therefore naturally do not enjoy paying, even when they have the money. Talk of money or payment arouses in most people negative emotions, even only for a brief moment. These negative emotions – no matter how minor or trivial – are the ones that the business savvy dentist who's bent on delivering the 9-Star Patient Experience must avoid at all costs.

The payment discussion is one definite opportunity for these negative emotions to be aroused in your patients. Your staff therefore, cannot afford to make the mistake of discussing payment right before the patient leaves. This avoids the possibility of having patients leave with a negative emotional experience.

Fred Joyal – one of the most eminent authorities on dental marketing – teaches that the question of payment must always be presented upfront because people's experiences are mostly colored by the event that aroused their emotions last. So, having the payment discussion upfront ensures it is not the last thing the patient hears before they leave, thereby preventing that discussion from arousing the last emotion they have – which will likely be negative.

Like I mentioned above, this ensures any negative thoughts that might arise in the patient's mind as a result of losing their prized possession, are dissolved way before the patient heads out of the door.

When payment issues have been discussed and done with, the patient continues on her treatment journey as you and your team bombard her with multiple moments of magic. When it's time for her to leave, your team sends her on her way with one of the most positive sendoff experiences of your team's choosing.

OFFER TO CHARGE THEIR DEVICES

MAKE THEM FEEL YOU CARE ABOUT THEM TOO MUCH BY OFFERING TO CHARGE THEIR GADGET

Like Dr. David Moffet always says, the delivery of a world-class service comes down to a series of magical moments that all combine to give the ultimate patient experience. It's the sum total of all the individual demonstrations of care that will reduce your patients' fear of dentistry and convince them to accept treatment now, as opposed to later.

A simple, but very effective demonstration of care is to offer to charge a patient's cellphone or other device while they undergo treatment.

While chances are high that most people who come in for a dental appointment will have phone chargers in their cars, having one of your staff offer to charge their phone or tablet shows that you are thinking about what matters to them. And having a fully charged phone matters to every living human.

Try it out and see how much people appreciate this gesture of care. You will be surprised how many people will take you up on the offer. And because very few, if any, service providers are thoughtful enough to do this, you will have given this patient something remarkable to talk about when they leave.

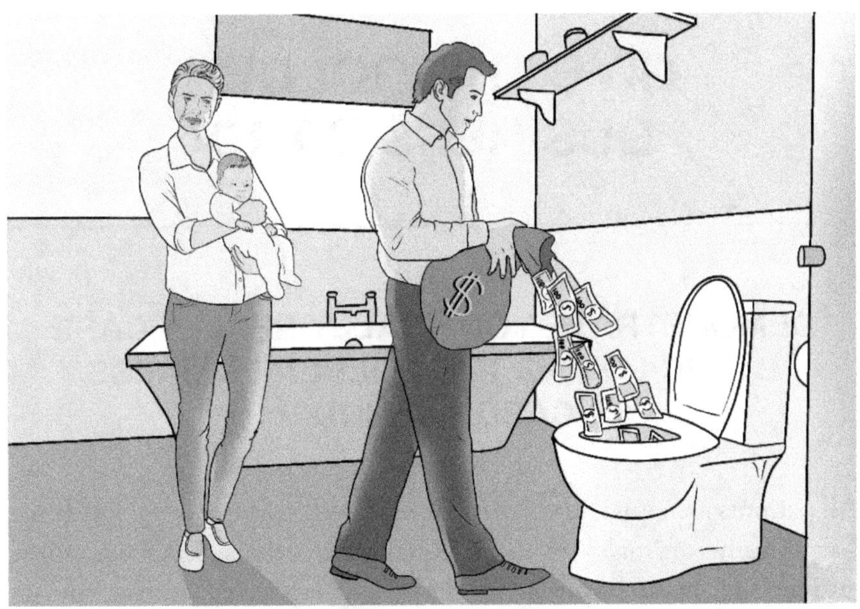

Fig 9: Are You Flushing Money Down The Toilet?

Without focusing on giving your current patients a 9-Star Experience, it won't matter what you spend your money doing to attract new patients… the results would be the same as those you would get were you to flush that money down the toilet. Go try it and see the result.

GIVE THE GOLDEN BUSINESS CARD

DEMONSTRATE YOU REALLY REALLY CARE BY DEPLOYING THE GOLDEN BUSINESS CARD METHOD[11]

All patients are equal, but like George Orwell said in his book Animal Farm, some animals are more equal than others. Likewise, some patients are more important than others; especially, to the bottom line. Patients who come in for higher value procedures that might result in serious pain or discomfort deserve an extra layer of VIP Treatment over and above the awesomeness dished out to everybody else.

This is how you go over and above to delight patients whose procedures might result in them suffering from pain or extreme discomfort when they leave your office. Have a special, very high-quality golden business card done for you. On it have your cellphone number and a special email address. Now here is where the moment of magic unfolds.

After the procedure with potential post-op pain or discomfort is performed, you hand out this special business card to the patient with the instruction to call you directly on the special number on the card or send you an email. Now… chances are very slim that patients will actually call you, but if they do, you answering that call will put you in a special group of very trusted people in the patient's life.

What handing out of that card does is demonstrate to the patient that you care. 87% of customers who switch service providers do so because they feel the service providers are indifferent. The reason I switched dental offices at the end of 2019 is because the people at the previous office didn't care.

GIVE THEM THE RED-CARPET TREATMENT

TREAT THE PATIENT TO A VIP RED CARPET EVENT

Do you perform high-value procedures like implants or other cosmetic dentistry? Do you want your practice to become a powerful magnet for high-value patients seeking these procedures? If your answer is yes – as it should be – then the following strategy is one you want to pay close attention to.

See, the idea behind driving the patient experience into the stratosphere is to take a page out of the Oscars red carpet experience and deploy it for patients that are coming in for high value procedures. So, let's say a patient is coming in to have implants done. This is how you wow the heavens out of them.

Engage the services of a Limousine company. Instruct the Limo service to arrive at the patient's house maybe 30 minutes prior to leaving. Also engage the services of a photographer and videographer to give the patient that all too familiar paparazzi experience.

Now, have a red carpet laid out from the Limo right up to the patient's front door. When the patient is ready to leave, have your videographer record her and photographs taken as she gets into the Limo. Have the Limo service provide the patient with a world-class service as she makes the trip to your office. (I can see Mrs. Peters' neighbors all standing by their front porches with cellphones recording the whole thing while wondering what on earth their neighbor is up to)

All this time, the Limo driver should be in constant contact with your office, so that your entire team is ready when the celebrity arrives. When Mrs. Peters arrives, have the red carpet rolled out from the Limo to your practice door. Give her the full-scale white glove service when she arrives and have your team ready her for the procedure. Once the procedure is done, treat the patient to the same VIP treatment as she makes her way into the Limo and back home.

Now…some people will say this is over the top and I agree. It is over the top. But if somebody is paying $5,000 or more for a procedure then what is $300 towards making their experience ultra-remarkable? This is marketing cost that you can write off at tax time, but even if you couldn't write this investment off, the other benefits make the extravagance worth it.

Imagine if some nosy news agency were somehow told of this event? They might not show up the first time they get notified. They might not up the second time, but the third or fourth time, somebody is going to show up with a real news camera. Imagine what would happen if your practice were to be on the evening news doing this?

Let's forget about the news people for a minute. How do you think the patient who has been treated to the life of a celebrity feel before, during, and after the procedure? Do you think she will be telling each and every one of her friends who she knows require the same procedure? You bet! This will be a major highlight of her LIFE. This is the stuff upon which VIP Smile Clubs are born.

Now… do you think the average dentist is going to do this? Hell no! And do you think your practice will be in the same class as any other dentists in your city? Absolutely not. Your practice will be in a category of its own and when you pull off stunts like these for the benefit of your patients, you can charge any price you wish.

THE DISCOUNTED CAR WASH

SURPRISE YOUR PATIENT WITH THE CHOICE OF HAVING A FREE CAR WASH

One of the tricks to delivering the 9-Star Experience is your practice developing relationships with service providers around you for the purposes of finding ways to wow your patients. Let's say your practice is close to a touchless, drive-through car wash facility. So you make arrangements with the facility to give your patients discounts as you will be sending them on a regular basis.

Here is how you create the moment of magic. During patient check-in, have your Front Desk team let the patient know that this week you are offering complimentary discounted car wash to all patients. It takes less than 10 minutes for a vehicle to go through touchless car wash, so most patients would take you up on this offer.

This is what this does. It adds an extra moment of magic to your service. If it were my dentist or chiropractor who did this to me, I would be thinking…holy cow, these people do go to great lengths to impress me.

Most humans are drawn to those who go to great lengths to treat them well. So, when you increase your prices or recommend a treatment, it's a combination of these magical moments that work to reduce resistance.

THE BIRTHDAY SURPRISE

WOW THEM WITH A MILESTONE BIRTHDAY SURPRISE.

People who like you will send a happy birthday message on social media if they don't miss the Facebook notification that today is your 40th, 50th or some other milestone birthday. People who say they love you on the other hand, will call you to wish you many more.

People who really love and care for you will, however, act differently. They will go a few steps further than send you a birthday message or card. They will do things on your birthday that demonstrate that they think about you and really want you to live longer and in good health. As a dental practice looking to demonstrate that you care, here is how you create a moment of magic out of a patient's milestone birthday.

One week before the milestone birthday, send them a birthday card with a well-thought-out message. You can have your entire team sign the card or have one person on your team do it. Inside the card include a stand-alone leaf/card message from you informing the patient that you have a birthday present for them at the office. Invite them to come and pick up the present during their birthday week.

The present does not need to be an expensive one at all, but it has to be meaningful. It can be a gift card, a book, a bottle of wine or anything you or your team chooses.

Now think about this…how many dental clinics have you seen or heard of that send or give real birthday gifts to their patients? And how do you think this action will make the patient feel? Do you think the patient will be talking about this to his or her friends and family? Do you think the patient will feel an obligation to keep her appointments? You bet they will. 100%.

Fig 10: Focusing On The Wrong Things?

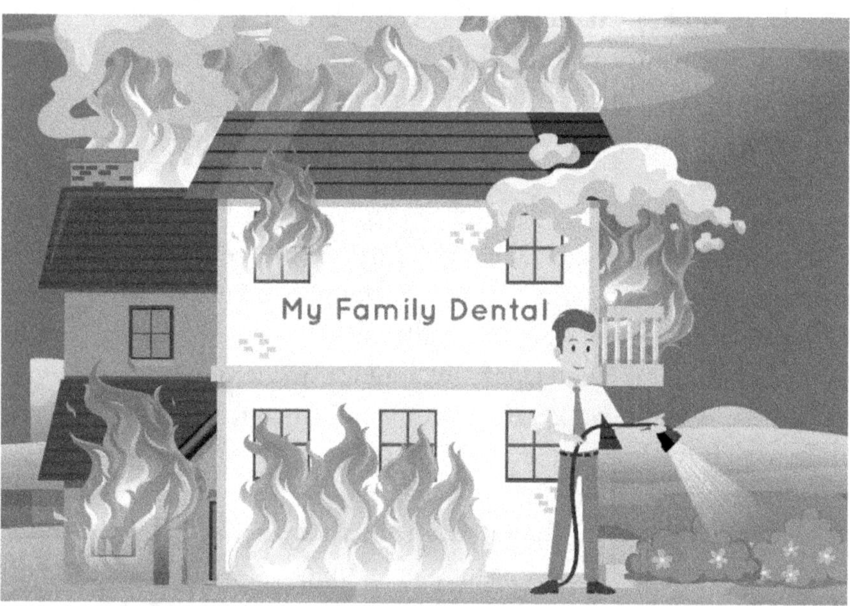

If you're not focusing on giving your patients the 9-Star Experience, you're focusing on the wrong things. Like the home owner who waters his flowers while his house is on fire.

ASK AFTER THEIR LOVED ONES...BY NAME

REMEMBER THEIR LOVED ONES' NAMES AND FIND WAYS TO MAKE SMALL TALK INVOLVING THEM

My wife and I moved to Calgary from Fort McMurray in 2017. Like all new residents in a city, we needed a Chiropractor. Having grown up poor in Zimbabwe, seeing a Chiropractor is not something my family did. In fact, I didn't know that such a Doctor existed until my late 20s. But my wife's story is different.

Even though she grew up in almost similar circumstances, her mom was a nurse, so she knew the importance of getting checked by every kind of doctor under the sun. So, she had us registered at Northern Hills Chiropractic. She and the kids did several massage and chiro sessions before she threatened to read the riot act to me if I didn't go see the Chiropractor. Apparently, my back issues were affecting my performance in the bedroom, so I really had no choice in the matter. So, I went.

After checking me in, the lady at the front desk said something that surprised me. She asked how Loice was doing. Yes, she asked how my wife was doing and used her first name while pronouncing it the way my mother-in-law wants her daughter's name pronounced. I was impressed. Not just by the fact that the front desk lady cared enough to ask after my wife's health, but by the fact that she remembered her name. Or did she? Or she used the tool at her disposal, her patient management software that had me as Loice's spouse? But that's beside the point.

The point is this. I felt great. That the front desk lady might have seen my relationship in her system never came to my mind. All I felt was this wuzzy feeling of goodness from thinking my wife must have done a great job of making an impression to these people so much that they still remember her name. Now, if this story had ended there, I would still have loved the experience, but it didn't. The awesomeness continued.

When my turn came, I went in to see the doctor. As I laid on the treatment table and did what the young doctor instructed, I wondered if I would be coming back. See, I sadly belong to the class of humans with a very low Chiropractic IQ, much the same way lots of people have a low Dental IQ. So, if nothing is visibly malfunctioning with my skeletal structure, I'm not coming in to see the Chiropractor. So, as I laid there being twisted and turned, I finally decided that I wasn't coming back anytime soon. But that decision changed in a flash.

As the Chiropractor told me I was done and instructed that I need to come and see him again in a few weeks, he said something that has had me coming in to see him more times than I care to admit. Now what did the young Asian doctor say that not only made me come back for his services, but also got me evangelizing on his behalf? Not to mention the number of times I've told this story… including writing it in this book.

This is what he said, word-for-word: "*How is young Divine's foot doing?*" Now, I don't know about you, but when a doctor enquires about your three-year-old child's foot — the mom had brought Divine as the boy was complaining his foot hurt – using the child's name, your relationship with that doctor changes. He or she ceases to be your doctor at that point. He or she becomes a family friend.

This is what I wish for your dental practice. For your patients to consider you a great family friend. Because when you get the status of being a family friend, your case acceptance goes through the roof, your referrals generation skyrocket, your reputation becomes magnetic, and your appointment cancellations drop like an iron ball.

HANG THEM ON THE WALL OF FAME

THIS STRATEGY WILL MAKE YOUR REFERRING PATIENTS FEEL RECOGNIZED, APPRECIATED, AND HIGHLY VALUED

One of the reasons why patients cancel appointments, develop no loyalty to a service provider, are not motivated to refer and don't bother reappointing is this…they just don't feel appreciated.

A good friend of mine moved to Toronto from Edmonton with his family of four. Knowing the atrocious indifference demonstrated by the dental office his family patronized in Edmonton, he and his wife decided to register at two separate dental offices. They did this so they could pick the one where the customer service was better.

Do you know the reason why they decided to have the entire family of five humans become patients at the office where the husband registered? Appreciation. And get this, it wasn't appreciation shown to the husband the first time he got there. It was appreciation shown to others by the dental office.

See, the practice where the husband registered for his free consultation had a large physical board on one wall of the waiting lounge titled: PATIENTS' WALL OF FAME. On the board were names of patients who had send referrals to the dental practice in the previous month. At the bottom of the board was a message that said…**We appreciate you talking about us!**

So as my friend sat there looking at the names on the board, he came to this realization… If this dental office goes as far as creating a wall of fame to appreciate and recognize people who send them referrals, chances are great they don't take their patients for granted as was the case at the last practice in Edmonton.

Five years later, my friend and his family have been happy clients at this practice in Toronto. And they have referred friends and colleagues who in turn have done the same. And their names have been up on the Wall of Fame several times.

Every major sport has its Hall of Fame where its greatest achievers are memorialized. Setting up a Wall of Fame to recognize and appreciate people that send referrals your way is a smart way to reward your patients. Set yours up!

NEVER FUMBLE THEIR NAMES

THE SAVVY DENTIST'S SECRET TO MAKING PATIENTS FEEL VALUED AND CARED FOR...

My first name is Farai. Most likely, you've never heard that name before, but you might have seen or heard of names like Fara or Farah, or Faraj. Now, this has happened to me on a few occasions when a doctor or some other professional has called me Farah or Faraj. Sometimes I correct them, sometimes I don't, but this annoys me every time. It's just a five-letter word. How hard can that be to remember? Especially, for somebody as smart as a doctor.

Have you ever forgotten a patient's name and in the process destroyed the treatment acceptance rapport that you and your team members had worked hard to build up to that moment when you fumbled the ball by calling Mrs. Jones Mrs. James?

And just so you know, which I think you do already... On the scale of major annoyances, few things rank higher than having your name said wrong. So, if you want to never forget your patient's name as you perform their procedure, here is the strategy Dr. Moffet and his team used to make sure the doctor never forgot the patient's name during treatment.

Here is what you do.

As part of your office's procedures, have your dental assistant or hygienist write the name of each patient in large visible letters on a post-it note just as the patient sits in the chair to have their treatment. Other valuable bits of information can also be included on the post-it note. Like the date of next appointment, children's names, an upcoming birthday, etc

As the patients gets settled into her chair, the assistant sticks the post-it note on the patient's bib, near their shoulder where the patient does not see it. [12]

Now…as you get to do your work, the patient's name and other valuable conversation starters are right there in front of you. With the patient's name staring at you like that, there is no way you can ever forget or bungle it. Including other pieces of information on the note dramatically improves your conversations and builds the type of trust that puts an end to future cancelled appointments and an increased case acceptance rate.

Once the treatment is complete, you bring their chair up and you gently lift off the post-it note. With confidence and authority, you proceed to thank the patient, wish her son a happy birthday and tell her that you look forward to seeing her again in December for her next cleaning or checkup.

This amazing demonstration of care and attention to detail is what makes patients feel valued and cared for. This is what makes patients feel like you are invested in their wellness. It is also what makes people accept your treatment recommendations and finally, it's this kind of care and attention to detail that will see your practice thrive in the unforgiving post-Coronavirus economy even when most other offices are being slaughtered.

BRING IN THE PATIENT WITH RESPECT

HOW TO BRING INTO THE TREATMENT ROOM PATIENTS WHOSE TIME HAS COME TO BE SEEN

Do you want to make your patients feel like real VIPs? Do you want to have the reputation of having Front Desk staff that brings out the feeling of being valued in your patients? If you do – as you certainly must – then this Moment of Magic will knock your socks off.

Imagine you are at a medical service office. You're sitting in the lounge waiting your turn to see the Doctor. As you pass time checking email, Facebook, and news on your phone, suddenly your name gets shouted by a lady standing by the door to the consultation rooms, holding a clipboard. "Emily Jones!"

If you're like most people, you are used to this sort of thing, so you shove your phone in your pocket or bag and follow the lady to the consultation room. That's the first experience. Now consider the following experience.

You're at another medical office sitting your turn to see the Doctor. As you do your thing on your phone, one of the Front Desk ladies approaches you. She stops 6 feet in front of you to observe some good social distance hygiene and greets you by name announcing that it's your turn to see the doctor. She motions for you to follow her and leads you to your consultation room.

Now…what's the difference between how you were treated at the two offices? At the first office, your name was shouted out in a room with three or four other people. No respect. Total indifference. In the other, you were respectfully approached and informed your turn had arrived in a way that demonstrated you matter.

How do you make your patients feel like VIPs even during such a simple activity as announcing their turn to see the doctor? Simple, let's borrow a page out of Dr. David Moffet's playbook.

First, you furnish your Front Desk Team with a printed schematic of your Waiting Lounge. If you want to take this a step further, you can upload the waiting room layout onto an iPad or Tablet.

As a patient sits down to wait his or her turn to be seen, a Front Desk team member takes note of where the patient sits, and marks this down on the schematic, along with the name and what the patient is wearing.

When it's time for the patient to come in for their consultation, the Front Desk team member responsible for ushering the patient to the treatment room looks at the schematic, identifies the patient on the diagram, walks out to the waiting room, greets them by name and informs them it's their turn to come in.

Now, if you want to treat your patients with class, this is how you do it. Greeting them personally, quietly, and directly as opposed to having their names shouted out the way it's done at the auction house.

GIVE THEM A TASTE OF VIP SPA TREATMENTS

DELIVERING THE VIP SPA EXPERIENCE TO DISSOLVE THE FEAR OF DENTISTRY AND GETTING PEOPLE TO TAKE TREATMENT NOW

Talk about launching the dental patient experience to the 9th Star… When Dr. David Moffet (author of *How to Build the Dental Practice of Your Dreams: (Without Killing Yourself!) in Less Than 60 Days)* was still running his practice in Sydney, Australia, one of the most magical of moments for their patients came when they were treated like VIPs at a luxury spa.

This is what Dr. Moffet and his team did. They invested in top of the line, individually packaged, heatable, moist towels. Each towel cost them a bank-busting 57 cents after getting them in packages of 1,000. He then invested in a small, good quality microwave oven (cost $58) and placed one in each treatment room.

Here is where the magic was created. At the end of a patient's appointment, one of these moist towels was warmed up and as soon as it reached a nice temperature, the towel was placed on a clean platter and handed over to the patient.

Now… if you've ever been to an upscale spa, flown first class or eaten in a high-end restaurant, then you've probably experienced this. Or you've seen it on TV or in the movies.

If you have ever experienced this level of service, you know that this is a seriously soothing and calming experience. One that will always be remembered and talked about by the patient for a long time to come. According to Dr. Moffet, it is an understatement to say that his patients looked forward to this experience. They could not wait to come back for more. Having one's mouth open for however long it takes to perform a procedure is not comfortable. Treating your patients at the end of procedures to a warm moist towel to sooth the face shows that you care.

The joy that your patients will experience during this moment of magic will put an end to cancelled future appointments. It will also drive your referrals through the roof and generate a tonne of 5-Star reviews for your practice. Besides these benefits, this experience also solidifies the patients' loyalty to your practice and places an iron fence around them against competing practices and priorities.

SECTION 2

YOUR OFFICE'S PERSONALITY

DITCH THE HOSPITAL SMELL

WHO ELSE WANTS TO GET RID OF THE HOSPITAL SMELL IN THEIR DENTAL OFFICE?

Very few people enjoy the smell of a hospital. As a species that seeks to survive and perpetuate itself, anything that is associated with insuring against our demise carries with it negative emotions. Visiting places where healthcare services are delivered rank at the top of things we do to prevent our demise. Necessary as they are, hospitals remind us of our mortality, and as a result, anything associated with them evokes negative emotions.

Top of the things that easily bring memories, thoughts, and feelings of being at a hospital or clinic is the smell. The hospital smell is unmistakable in both its identity and effect on the negative emotions it arouses.

As a business savvy dentist, the last thing you want is for people to experience in your practice the same smell they experience when they visit a hospital. Most people want to get well when they are sick, but that's as much as we want to be close to anything that smells like a hospital.

In the post-Coronavirus era, people have used so much hand sanitizer that the only memory that hand sanitizer elicits is the depressing feelings and anxiety they felt during the pandemic. This is not the kind of smell you want your patients to experience as they come in and get treatment in your office. So, how do you ensure your patients experience the most calming and uplifting smells while in your office?

Do what Dr. Nouri at Thousand Oaks Dental Spa does. Give your patients aromatherapy.[13] If you do not want to give aromatherapy as part of your package, then invest in some form of scent circulation system for the entire practice.

If you get into any upscale establishment, you will always be greeted with an aroma that is part of the mystique of that establishment. This is true at the Ritz, the Four Seasons or any such establishment where customer experience is front and center of the business strategy.

So, ask yourself this…how well thought out is your office aroma? What do people think when they experience the smell of your practice? If there was an anxiety-measuring device that tracked people's anxiety on a scale of 1 – 10 based on the how close to a hospital smell your dental practice's scent is, where would your office rating fall? Ask your team what they think and act on their answers. Also ask your patients and get them involved. Not only does it make them feel good to know that you care what they think, asking the patients themselves also gives you their unfiltered opinion on this very important subject.

MAKE THE PATIENT FEEL CALM

MAKING PATIENTS FEEL CALM AND AT EASE DURING TREATMENT

Being an oral health expert, you know more than most other health experts that anxiety is one of the most insidious factors that stops people from coming in to see you as often as they ought to.

For you, the most serious disservice the Coronavirus pandemic has done is to exponentially increase your patients' level of anxiety when it comes to seeking your services. Unless it's an emergency, most people will not be making dental appointments in a hurry. Most people's anxiety has them in a state of waiting to see how things improve before they commit to booking an appointment.

So, when a patient comes in, you must give them such an anxiety-busting experience that they will go talk about it to everybody in their world. You want people to feel at home in your chair so that they not only return, but also refer and encourage their friends and loved ones to come in and see you.

Some of the best ways to reduce patient anxiety is to emulate what Dr. Nouri at Thousand Oaks Dental Spa is doing. A patient can watch a movie on Netflix with noise-cancelling headphones and is covered with a warm blanket and her head resting on warm pillow while her hands are covered with paraffin. To ensure maximum privacy, the curtains are shut, and the lights are turned low.

After a dental visit, patients come out feeling pampered and refreshed, something that you would not normally experience at the dentist. This is the kind of experience that makes for viral social media posts that will get a flood of both new and current patients coming in to see you. And the last time I checked, a flood of patients is a good problem to have for a dental practice at a time when many practices are finding it hard to find their footing after the Coronavirus brought the entire world to a grinding halt.

Fig 11: Viral Patient Experience

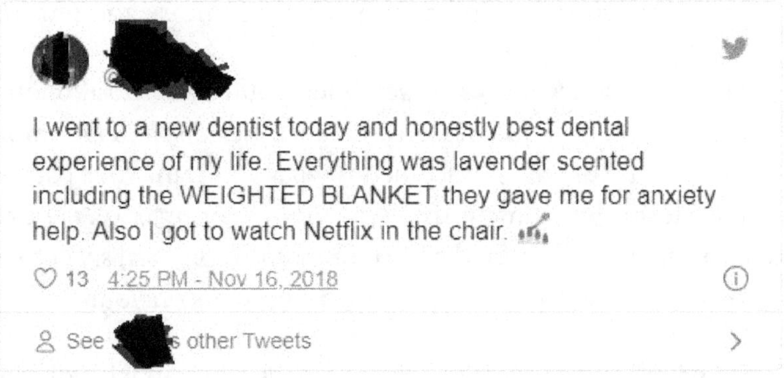

SAY NO TO ANXIETY-INSPIRING WALLS

WHAT'S THE WRITING ON YOUR WALLS?

In an era when people are always on guard and tense – no thanks to the Covid-19 pandemic – the last thing you want is to have your physical space contribute to patients' sense of unease and tension.

Think of the feeling you'd get when you enter into the lobby of a Ritz-Carlton, The Four Seasons, or an upscale spa. The ambiance and warm feeling of being welcomed is what you want your patients to experience from the moment they set foot in your practice. One of the most important elements that contribute to your physical space's feeling of welcome and warmth is the pictures and posters on your walls.

So, what's on your walls? Are your walls adorned with disgusting photos of decayed teeth? Or do you have images of diseased gums or gaping mouths with missing teeth staring at patients as they sit in the waiting lounge? If you do, it's time to take them down. It does not help that these unpleasant images have beside them great looking after-images of gleaming and perfect teeth.

The damage done by nasty-looking before photos is irreversible, so please take them down. Unless of course… if your goal is frightening the crap out of your patients to the point of making them so tense and uncomfortable that they resist and tune out anything you and your team say. I doubt very much that is your goal. So, what do you do?

Invest in tasteful paintings and portraits that inspire comfort and contribute to creating the ambiance of warmth and comfort that you want your patients to experience. Like I said above, the last thing you want is to increase the tension felt by patients who are already in a state of perpetual tension and anxiety as a result of everything that's been going on in the world. Make a deliberate decision to put images that inspire and make people comfortable.

Fig 12: Are You Shooting Yourself In The Foot?

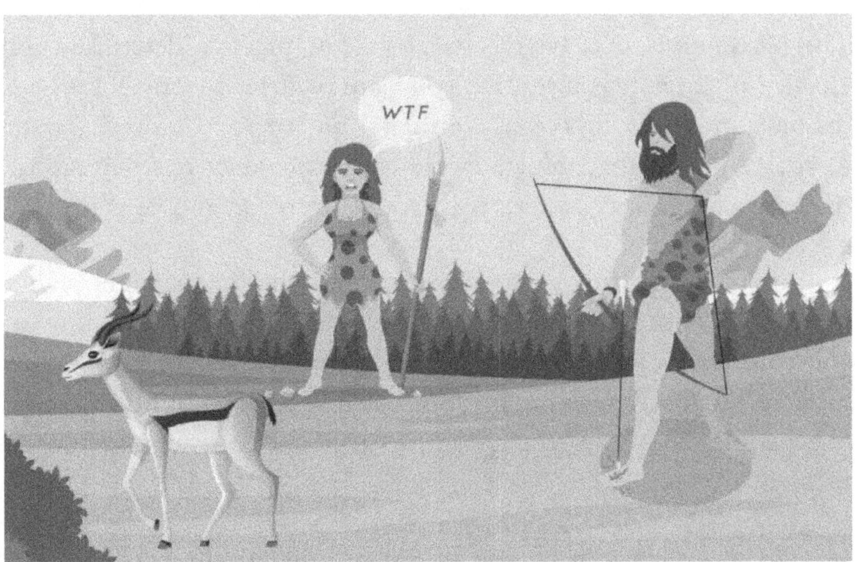

Having posters and other images that drive up your patients' discomfort and anxiety is driving your case acceptance down. It's like the hunter who points the arrow at his leg instead point it at the deer.

Moment of Magic #22

UPGRADE YOUR BEVERAGES

BUILD UP THE PERCEPTION OF HIGH VALUE BY UPGRADING YOUR BEVERAGES

The perceptions that people have of your practice determine the 'quality' of patients you get. Do you want to attract people for whom the only and most important consideration is price? Or do you want to attract people that value a world-class experience over and above the basic clinical service they will receive from you and your team?

Doing those things that attract people who value a high-quality experience is not only good for the bottom line. It's also good for you and your team's mental health. Cheap people are a pain in the butt to serve. Anybody who has been in business for two minutes knows that people who want to pay as little as possible are a real pain the [expletive].

So, what else can you do to not only create the perception of quality and luxury, but also to deliver it in your dental practice? Here is a simple but amazingly effective way high end spas do it. Just replace cheap water with a high-end brand like Evian or Perrier.

When I'm offered a bottle of cheap water or when cheap bottles of water are stocked in the fridge at a dentist or some other service provider, I accept, but that's the end of it. If I don't finish the water before my visit, I leave the half full bottle or just throw it in the trash as soon as I leave.

However, not the case with a high-end brand of water like Evian or Perrier. No sir! That one I make sure I don't finish so that I can take it with me. It's a status symbol to be seen walking in the grocery store holding a bottle of Evian water in my hand. Yes, I know what you're thinking, and I agree. I'm vain. But so are millions of other humans.

As I take slow sips of that water (and most of us make sure to consume the water in public), I'm subconsciously thankful to whoever has given me this symbol of high living, because I know other people notice.

Now I know some people will say, well, it's just water. To which I'll add the correction that it's not just water. It's Evian water or to put it in the words of one good friend, it's Perrier. The subconscious thought that it was my dentist's office that gave me the water will not be lost on me when it comes to considering a treatment recommendation, or when I start debating whether or not I should cancel my cleaning appointment and reschedule for 10 years from today.

So, take a look at the kind of beverages that you're offering your patients. If you're offering stuff that's on the cheap side, please consider getting an upgrade. Investments in quality always pay off.

BREAK BREAD WITH YOUR PATIENTS

USING THE HUMAN LOVE OF BUILDING RELATIONSHIPS OVER FOOD TO MAKE YOUR PATIENTS FEEL LIKE THEY JUST VISITED AN OLD FAMILY FRIEND[14]

What do you do when a good friend visits your home? If you're a great host – which I've heard and also seen on social media that you are – you already know how they like their tea, coffee or drink of choice. So, you make it and give them. You don't even need to ask.

What about a new friend whom you've just met and would like to develop a deeper relationship with? What do most awesome people do to deepen a new promising relationship? You most likely invite them for dinner, lunch, drinks, or just coffee at the good old Starbucks.

Why? What is it about sharing a meal, a beverage or drink that brings humans closer? I won't pretend to be a social anthropologist with an answer to this, but this I will say with confidence. Humans have been bonding over food and drink for millennia. Sharing a meal or drink with somebody says I care about you; I feel safe around you and I'm comfortable in your presence.

Now, if you want your dental patients to feel comfortable and to develop a deeper bond with your practice (the kind old friends have for each other), create a moment of magic involving you or your team member sharing coffee or tea with the patients. Here is how it's done.

Have one of your team members offer tea or coffee to the waiting patient or patients like this.

"Mrs. Brown and Mr. Jones, I'm just about to go out to grab myself a Chai Latte at Starbucks. What can I get for you while you wait for Dr. Chen?"

Said like this, your team member has removed the feeling or thought inside the patient's mind that they might be inconveniencing the team member by having them get the beverage for them since the team member was going to get their own beverage anyway.

If you have a regular self-serve coffee maker inside your office – as most practices do these days – consider investing in a touchless coffee machine that patients do not touch or hold to pour the beverage. People are reluctant to use anything that others can touch, no thanks to Covid-19.

As a patient leaves the front desk to take her seat in the waiting lounge, have one of the team members make the offer in the way described above and watch the patient's level of comfort go through the roof while their anxiety drops to the floor.

Now… how many dentist's offices have you been to where patients get served with a beverage of their choice in this way. In most offices, a member of the front desk just says, *"help yourself to a coffee there Mr. Brown."* No finesse, no tact, total indifference.

SECTION 3

THE DIGITAL EXPERIENCE

Fig 13: Is Your Digital Presence Sleeping On the Job?

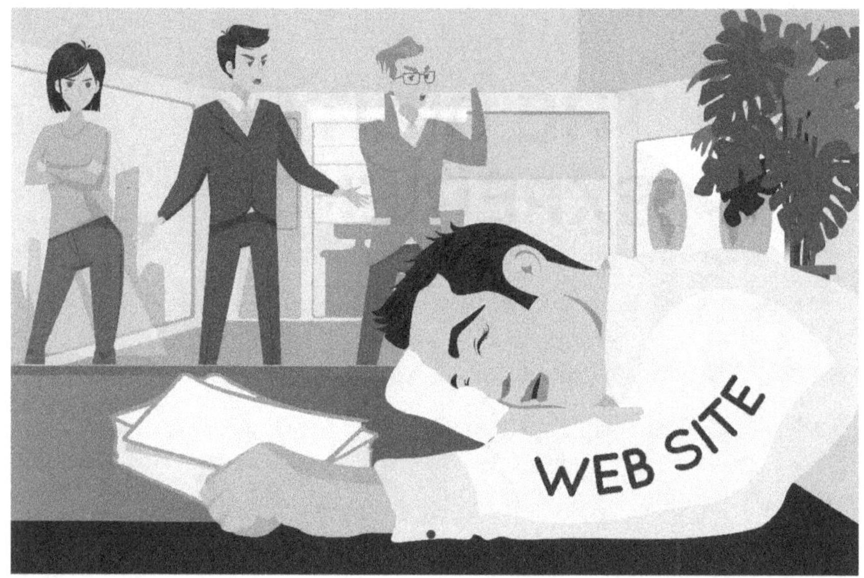

Is your presence online helping you or it is like
a front desk employee who is asleep at the desk
while patients wait in frustration to served?

Moment of Magic #24

BE FRIENDLY...
ON ALL DEVICES

CREATE A POSITIVE EXPERIENCE WHEN PEOPLE INTERACT WITH YOUR BRAND ACROSS ALL DIGITAL DEVICES

Few digital experiences are as frustrating as trying to navigate, a website on a mobile phone, that's not been optimized for mobile devices. Given the fact that every adult who would be coming in to see you will most likely have a smart phone, one of the best digital experiences you can give your patients is having a fully mobile friendly website.

Your videos, images and formatting must work as good on an iPhone, a tablet, or a desktop computer. There must be no difference. Given that your website is a big part of the experience your patients have with your brand, it becomes mission critical to ensure you have a website that works as it should on digital devices.

Test your website today. Find out how it looks and works on a variety of devices. If something is not working right, then you have to get that fixed ASAP. Loosing patients to the competition because of a website that's not optimized to work on all devices is dumb. And you're not dumb. You're a Dentist.

DEVELOP A MAGNETIC DIGITAL PERSONA

HOW TO CREATE A DIGITAL PERSONA THAT MAKES PROSPECTS WANT TO COME INTO YOUR OFFICE IN PERSON TO SEE YOU

Dr. Tarun Agarwal, the driving force behind the extremely successful practice, Dental Arts in Raleigh, North Carolina was talking on the Dental Practice Heroes podcast[15] the other day when he mentioned something very poignant. He said by the time a patient decides on which dental office to call, he or she would have checked out several dentists on the web. Now… can you guess which page gets checked out the most?

If you said, it's the 'Meet The Doctor' page, you're absolutely right. So, to Dr. Agarwal's point, most new patients choose who to call based on the experience they have while interacting with the Dentist on the practice website. The importance of creating a welcoming persona on the web therefore becomes glaringly obvious when one considers that the Dentist's web or digital persona is first point of contact between a Dentist and his or her prospective new patients.

However, when one considers that most dentist personas on the web today are generic and average, you start to think the importance is not so obvious. Yet creating an effective persona is one of the lowest hanging fruits with which a dentist can create one of the most powerful emotional connections with his or her potential patients. I'm sure you know or have heard that people buy on emotions, and then use facts to justify their decisions. To create a digital persona that emotionally connects with your potential patients, so that they are compelled to take the next step by calling your office or booking an appointment, you must do the following.

Show pictures of yourself contributing to causes in the community. Let people see your family and how like them you are. Showcase your local and international charity work and even go as far as inviting people to join you. Show people the hobbies you enjoy and tell your story. Use the services of a good copywriter to present your educational qualifications in terms of how that education and training directly benefits the patients. On its own, the list of CE courses you've done through the years will not give people the digital experience that will pull them into your office. But presented in terms of how those courses translate into benefits for the patients, you'll have them itching to come in after seeing how educated you are.

Now…here is a word of caution. Please don't put pictures of your new BMW, Benz or pictures of you dropping your kids at the most expensive private boarding school in the country. Even more important, please do not put pictures of yourself posing besides a lion or giraffe you just shot, if this is your thing. You don't want to give people reasons to dislike you or to think that their money is going to fund your life of luxury…even if in reality, it does and should. (wink wink)

THE MAGNETIC DIGITAL WELCOME

HOW TO CREATE A DIGITAL EXPERIENCE THAT OFFERS A WELCOME EXPERIENCE THAT PULLS WEB VISITORS INTO YOUR OFFICE

Before people around the world were given stay-at-home orders to prevent the spread of the Coronavirus, many dental practices actually did ok financially even when they had a web/digital presence that repulsed people. They still did ok because people's reliance on the internet had not reached the proportions that were ushered in by the coronavirus instigated stay-at-home orders. Things are now different. Very different.

People now put a much higher premium on their digital experiences than they have ever done before. Yet a casual look on the web shows a plethora of dental websites all vying for the title of MRPE — Most Repulsive Patient Experience. Having invested large sums of money to attend dental school and in building their practices, I know most dentists deploy these repulsive web experiences unintentionally. They mean well. They just got bad advice.

Given your smarts, you must by now be wondering what it is about a dental practice's digital presence that gives patients a repulsive experience. Well, wonder no more and ask yourself this. *How much of your digital copy (web, social media, email and text message copy) talks about you and your practice compared to how much it talks about your patients and their challenges, desires, and fears?*

People develop bonds of trust and liking in those people who focus on them as opposed to those who focus themselves. Nobody enjoys the experience of being around somebody who talks about themselves all the time. So, is the copy/messages in all your digital assets centered around the aspirations, challenges and fears faced by your current and prospective patients? Or does it talk about how qualified you and your team are, what advanced equipment you have and how great you are?

Have you ever been in a conversation with somebody who talks him/herself and how good they are without giving you any chance to talk? How was that experience? If it was a first date, how far did that relationship go? Not very far I'd guess. So, if you and me are repulsed by the experience of interacting with a self-centered person, how do you think people feel when they get to your website, Treatment Page or Facebook page and all they read or listen to is you talking about yourself and your great practice? They also feel repulsed. Just as you would around a 'me-me' type person.

Do you want to find out whether or not your digital copy is you-centric or patient-centric? Do this quick test. Copy the block of text/copy on your website that you want to test for its *You vs. Patient* Centeredness. Paste the block of text/copy onto Perry Marshall's platform at <u>https://www.perrymarshall.com/grade/</u>. Click the button Check Text Readability. See Image overleaf.

If you talk about yourself more than you talk about your patients, then know that your digital presence is driving people away, and you must start working towards correcting that problem because like it or not, it's costing you money.

Using the Perry Marshall You vs. Them tool to test if web copy on my website, www.dentistryflywheel.com home page talks about you, our clients, more than it talks about ourselves. The piece of copy I tested talks about my clients 1.4 times more than it talks about me and my company. That is what you want your website copy to be in order for it not to be repulsive to visitors.

Fig 14: Is Your Web Copy Narcissistic?

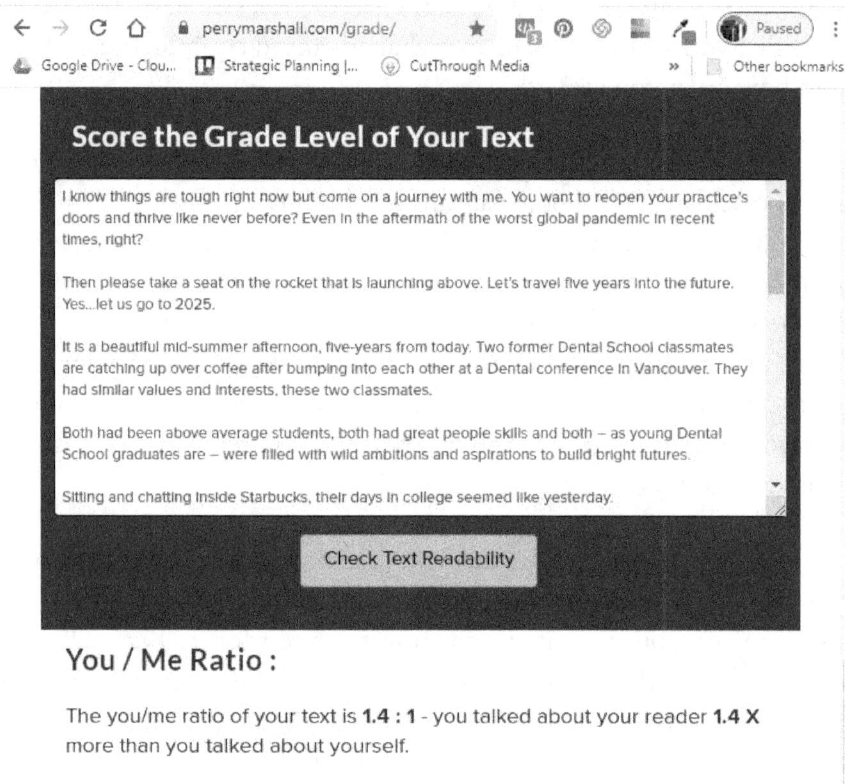

BE THEIR FAITHFUL GUIDE

GUIDE YOUR PROSPECTIVE PATIENTS TO YOUR OPERATORY CHAIRS BY GIVING THEM AN EMOTIONAL EXPERIENCE THAT'S BUILT AROUND A MARKETING FUNNEL

For the savvy dentist's patients – both current and prospective – to respond to his or her marketing strategy, a well-thought-out emotional pathway experience must be built for the benefit of the patient. This means as the patient interacts with your digital presence, she should be guided through the digital pathway towards two critical goals. First, to remove all anxiety and fear in the patient; and second, to get the case accepted and treatment provided.

The best way to execute the digital side of Case Acceptance (which as it stands, is the initial interaction most patients will have with your brand) is by employing The Dentistry Funnel. At its heart, The Dentistry Funnel Method acknowledges the fact that when you do your marketing, for that marketing to be effective, you must be targeting five distinct groups of people.

Group 1: People who see your advertising
Group 2: People who click the ads
Group 3: People who call your office
Group 4: People who book appointments
Group 5: People who accept treatment

For the people in these five groups to have a positive experience with your marketing, the marketing messages must:

1. Be targeted specifically to each group
2. Be so designed only to move the prospect to the level below
3. Each group may need its own channel of execution. (People who see your ads will do so on Facebook or Instagram and they will see your offer and call to action on your Treatment Landing Page.)

Besides giving your prospective patients an experience with which to build trust in you, one other benefit that comes with deploying your marketing within a Dentistry Funnel is the ability for you to track and measure every activity within the funnel. With great tracking and measurement comes the ability to fine-tune the experience, all for the benefit of the patient and your bottom line. All the benefits that will accrue to your patients because you deployed the Dentistry Funnel Method will come because the method allows you to create and deploy an integrated marketing strategy.

Your call to action here, therefore, is to start thinking about transitioning your marketing into the Dentistry Funnel framework. The benefits to your practice will be self-evident in:

1. An excited patient base. You want your patients to be excited.
2. Marketing efforts that're easier to track and measure
3. Increased patient recall rates
4. Drastically declining appointment cancellations
5. Consistent in-flow of high-quality referrals
6. Consistent increase in the number of high-value procedures

Fig 15: The Dentistry Funnel

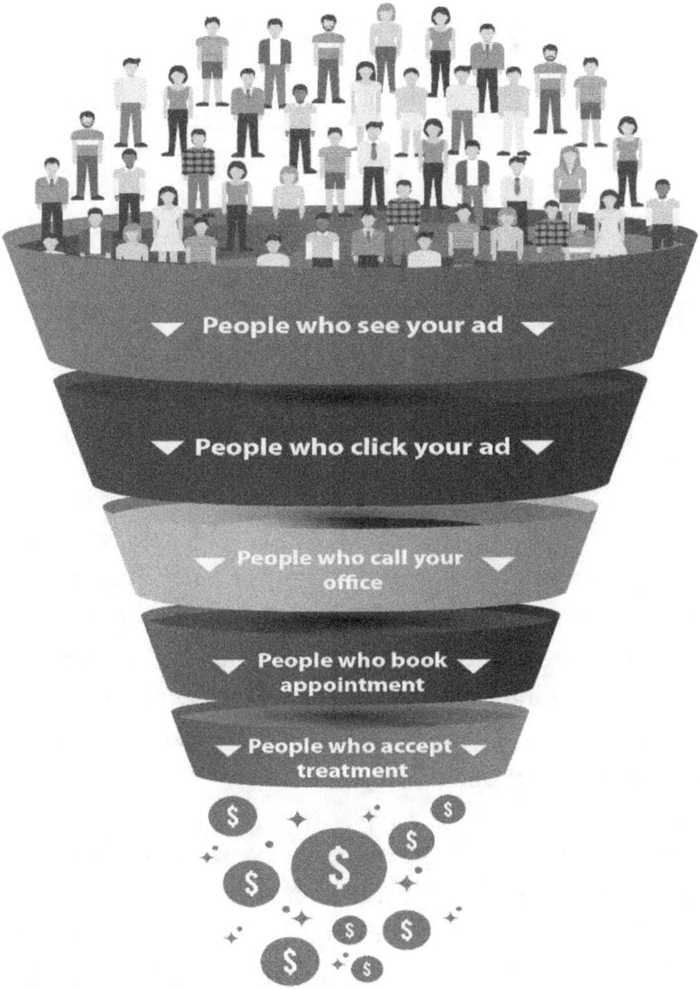

Moment of Magic #28

MAKE THEM ITCH TO GET YOUR OFFERS

HOW TO GIVE YOUR PATIENTS AN ADVERTISING EXPERIENCE THAT GETS THEM ITCHING TO KNOW MORE ABOUT YOUR TREATMENT OFFERS

Imagine you are on a first date. Everything is going great until your date-mate starts talking about where you will be going for your honeymoon, how he or she wants 3 kids with you, how he or she wants 2 dogs (one called Bingo and another called Ringo) and where your family will be going for vacations. What will be going through your mind before you find, as quickly as you can, the best excuse to run for your life? Granted, such an experience would traumatize you for life and you would pray the gods do not make you come close to a person like that ever again.

That is exactly what happens when a dentist puts out advertising that asks people to book a consultation right on the ad itself. Unless you haven't been looking, these kinds of ads with a call to action button that says 'Book Now' or 'Schedule an Appointment' are the staple on social media advertising platforms. By asking people who see the ad to book an appointment, the entire ad copy does the equivalent of asking for a hand in marriage right on the first date. And as you can guess, these ads don't work. Why?

Because they give prospective patients the same bad emotional experience one would get were they to be asked for marriage on the first date. This is the reason why most dental ads bring dismal results. Business savvy dentists do not do this. They understand that the best experience to give a prospect who sees their ad is to expose them to emotionally-charged ad copy that has just but one goal - to capture attention by creating curiosity. That curiosity is built to result in getting into the next stage of the Funnel by clicking the 'Learn More' button.

By just emotionally engaging your prospect at this early stage of your relationship, you begin the important work of making them trust you. It's these initial bonds of trust that form when the prospect is reading or watching your ad that will pull them into wanting to know more about you, your brand, and your offer.

So, as in a great date with a great person, you want your ad to be emotionally intriguing enough to have them asking or agreeing to a second date, which in the case of your dental ad, is having them click the call to action, taking them into the next stage of the funnel, which is the group of people who have clicked your ads.

Moment of Magic #29

MAKE THEM WANT TO KNOW MORE

HOW TO DELIVER A DIGITAL EXPERIENCE THAT GETS PROSPECTIVE PATIENTS WHO CLICK YOUR ADS ITCHING TO CALL OR BOOK AN APPOINTMENT

One of the biggest mistakes quite a lot of dentists make with their marketing is failing to think about the experience they desire for the prospective patients who've seen their advertising and clicked on them. Simply put, how do patients feel after landing on the next stage of your marketing funnel? When a person clicks your ad, where are they taken and what is their experience when they get there?

I have seen so many dental ads that when clicked, I ended up on a dental office's home page. And I have seen different versions of ads ending up on a single generic landing page. Haven't you seen ads for different procedures by one dental office on Facebook that when clicked, they all take you to the same form having only the practice logo, contact details and empty fields for you fill? I do not see how this rough experience would help in getting a prospective patient to fill the empty form fields and be excited to come in. If you know of one, please do let me know.

Savvy dentists who will thrive in the post Covid-19 world will thrive because they understand something those who struggle don't, and it is this…a random person who clicks their ad on Facebook or IG ceases to be a random human the moment they click the ad. This person becomes a potential patient – someone who has the potential to contribute towards a secure retirement and your children enjoying the best education money can buy. This person becomes a lead whose relationship with you from then on needs to be treated differently from the way a random pedestrian is treated.

The emotional pathway and experience that the person who clicks your ad goes through has to be thoughtfully crafted and strategically deployed. Sending paid traffic (potential patients) to a generic form or a website home page is neither thoughtful nor strategic. To be thoughtful and strategic in creating the most effective experience for your leads, you need to build and deploy Treatment Landing Pages for each procedure your practice does.

A Treatment Landing Page is a web page that's dedicated to a single procedure that your clinic offers. In many ways, it is the home page for the specific procedure you're advertising. As such, it should make visitors feel welcome, comfortable and identify with the treatment story theme. By using a powerful Story (video or text) of Transformation and emotionally rich copy, the Treatment Landing Page will guide your prospect towards one goal and one goal alone — to get your offer by either calling your office or booking an appointment.

To be successful in pulling the prospective patient into your office in person, the Treatment Landing Page must be built using the time-tested and proven principles of direct response marketing. Because they are an integral component of a Dentistry Funnel, Treatment Landing Pages have the ability to present the advertised treatment in a way that exponentially increases the chances of the patient booking an appointment to come in.

Again, this is all about giving the patient a digital experience that demonstrates you care by exposing them to the following elements of the Treatment Landing Page.

- ⇨ Emotional, attention-grabbing headline
- ⇨ A powerful video testimonial Story of Transformation
- ⇨ Emotional, benefits-driven copy/message
- ⇨ Trust-builder, Irresistible Offer, and a Call to Action
- ⇨ Scarcity driver and Social proof

Fig 16: Treatment Page Sample

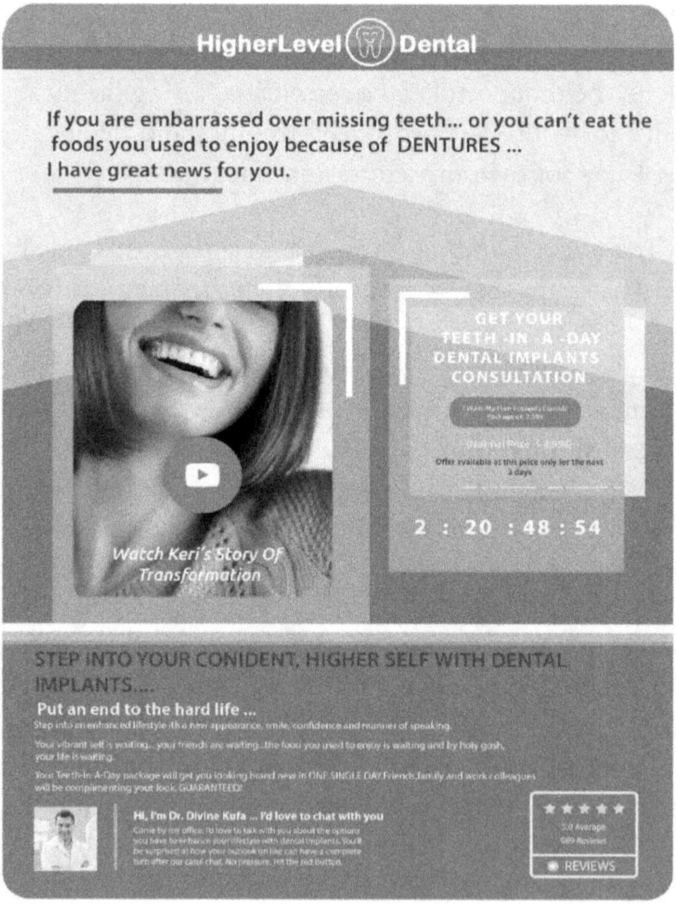

SECTION 4

THE COMMUNITY EXPERIENCE

GIVING BACK THAT ENDEARS YOU TO THE COMMUNITY

CREATE A COMMUNITY OF RAVING FANS USING DR. GARY TAKACS' STRATEGY...THE UPSIDE IN COLLECTIONS IS AMAZING[16]

I loved this strategy when I heard it on the Thriving Dentist podcast with Dr. Gary Takacs DDS, and dental marketing power broker, Naren Arulrajah. Given the fact that it's going to be a while before physical distancing regulations allow group community events to be done – no thanks to Covid-19 – implementing the community sports team Mouthguard Strategy is absolutely one of the best ways a savvy dentist can create a very profitable experience for his community. Here is how it works.

You make a small investment in materials and equipment – under $4000. You then identify a sports team within the community you operate in and you offer to make the team customized NFL quality mouthguards for free.

Getting parents, coaches, and school heads to agree is an easy sell, because every soccer, hockey, rugby, basketball, football or lacrosse parent wants their child's teeth protected. Now, if you are offering to give – for FREE – NFL quality mouthguards that are custom-made to fit their child's mouth, you have a no brainer on your hands when it comes to whether or not parents and the school will support the project.

To get you and your team going, you need to invest in materials and a suckdown machine. When he got started, Dr. Takacs invested $1000 for materials to make the mouthguards and got himself the Great Lakes Orthodontics thermo suckdown machine that cost him about $2,200. According to Dr. Takacs, this $3,200 investment resulted in $101,000 worth of dentistry in 2019 from the patients that came as a result of the mouth guard project.

Dr. Takacs involves his whole team and makes a whole event out of the entire process of bringing the team and their family members in to get their guards fitted up. He creates a Shock and Awe gift bag for the parents containing toothpaste, hand sanitizer, marketing material, toothbrushes, and other items of swag. Everything in the Shock and Awe bag is branded to his practice. Lastly, the gift bag will contain a letter of invitation for the recipient to join Dr. Takacs' practice.

Now, as far as benefits to the practice go – as demonstrated by Dr. Takacs' $101,000 boost in collections – this project will bring into your marketing orbit the team's parents, aunts, uncles, nieces, nephews, cousins, grandparents, the coaches and their families, faculty and all the alumni. If you ask me, this is a marketing grand slam.

The benefits for your practice are too many to go over one by one, but more than that, it's the multiple Moments of Magic created by the project for everybody involved. The buzz that will result out of this project might result in you suspending some external marketing because social media will be aflame with the story, the news media would love to have a piece of the action and the team itself and its family members will be forever grateful.

If you'd like to know more, you can check out the amazing Dr. Gary Takacs' The Thriving Dentist Podcast or program here at https://www.thrivingdentist.com/giveaway/. As of this writing, Dr. Takacs was giving the program training for free, so depending on when you'll be reading this book, the promotion might be over, but feel free to get in touch with him at https://www.thrivingdentist.com/.

Fig 17: Shooting Yourself In The Foot?

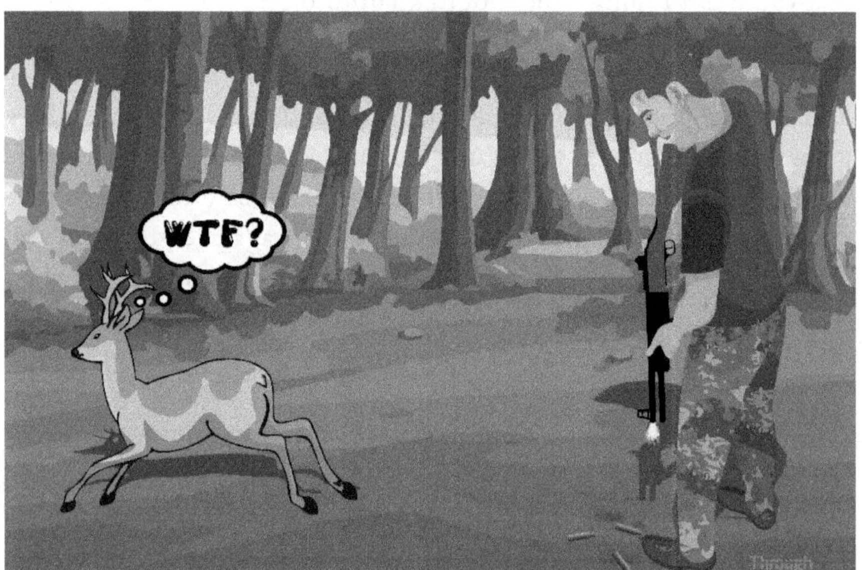

The dental practice that does not invest in the community it works in shoots itself in the foot. The positioning that comes with giving back and investing in the community you work in sets you up as the go-to dental office. It positions you as a practice that really cares for the community. Great things happen for the dental practice that's viewed as the most committed to the community.

SHOW LOVE ON YOUR PATIENTS' CLIENTS

HELP A PATIENT WHO'S IN BUSINESS CREATE A GREAT EXPERIENCE FOR THEIR OWN CLIENTS OR CUSTOMERS

Do you have in your patient base somebody who owns a business or who is in a top leadership position at his or her company? Just like you, your patients that are business owners or have leadership roles in business have clients of their own to whom they'd like to give some great experiences. How about you make some smart moves to help your business leader patients deliver an awesome experience to their own clients?

Imagine how a business leader you've just worked on will feel after you hand him two copies of a business book with instructions for him to give the other copy to a business leader friend or client of his? If this was me getting these two copies, I'd be thinking, *holy cow man, this dentist doesn't stop at thinking about me, she also thinks about my clients.* Not only would I make sure that I pass on this gift to a client, I would make sure the client knows it's a gift from my Dentist and highly recommend her.

Now… if you really want to become legendary, you will do this as a Pay-It-Forward Challenge in which you challenge whoever you're giving the books to do exactly the same thing you've done. Oh, did I mention that you could create a Facebook Page for the Challenge and watch it take a life of its own?

I can see the news headlines several months from now… *'Local Dentist starts a book challenge that has had 1000 books shared among the city's business elite.'* Now, if I was someone looking for a great dentist, this is the one I would be going to and it won't matter that I have to drive an hour to get to his office.

MAKE IT EASY FOR PEOPLE TO CHOOSE YOU

BECOME A TRUSTED AUTHORITY AND SOURCE FOR HELP IN YOUR COMMUNITY

Who do patients trust more amongst several Dentists - as they browse dental websites looking for a new Dentist - the one who has published a book on a dentistry subject, or one who hasn't?

Obviously, people will trust the authority on a subject and the authority is always the person who has written a book. The savvy dentist makes it super easy for people to pick him or her over every other dentist in the community by positioning him or herself as the authority.

Let me ask you this. Do you want to explode your Invisalign or Implants production with people flooding into your office because they FEEL they trust you? Do you want your case acceptance to go through the roof because you've made it super comfortable for people to trust your recommendations?

If your answer is yes – as it should be – then do what Adam Witty and Rusty Shelton instructed in their Amazon best seller, Authority Marketing. Write a book on the procedure you would like to build extreme trust in. By writing a book and handing out this book to your patients, you are validating their decision to have chosen you as their dentist.[17]

Imagine the impact on trust and comfort level your book will have on a patient browsing your website's home page. Like already mentioned somewhere in this book, people will check out several dental practices before they decide to call one. So why not set yourself apart by becoming the Dentist who wrote the book on Implants, Invisalign, Veneers, or Crowns?

Take a leaf out of the playbooks of some of the most successful Dentists. They are all published authors. Drs – Dustin Burleson, Paul Etchison, Anissa Holmes, Mark Costes, David Moffet, Howard Farran, Rinesh Ganatra and many others have all written books that have solidified their authority in their respective communities. Writing your book will take time and effort, but the effect on how much trust your patients will have in you will be well worth the investment.

INVEST IN THE COMMUNITY

GIVE BACK INTO YOUR COMMUNITY SO THAT YOUR PATIENTS KNOW THAT YOU'RE NOT THERE JUST TO TAKE THEIR MONEY...LIKE OTHERS DO

People do business with people they know, like, and trust. It takes time and effort to build a relationship that allows the bonds of knowing, trusting, and liking to develop. But when they are developed, the parties to that relationship will enjoy great things.

So how do you as a dentist create opportunities for your patients to develop a strong relationship with your practice? How are practices that are thriving getting this done? Pre-Covid-19, business savvy dentists sponsored events that did a lot to cement their position and relationship with their community. Events like soccer games, hockey games, summer BBQs and other community events were leveraged to create community experiences that led to practice growth.

Not anymore or anytime soon anyway. With physical distancing having become a central part of our new normal, group community events that savvy dental practices used to sponsor and leverage will not be possible in the foreseeable future. New ways of bringing the community together are needed.

So, while group events won't be an experience accessible for all communities, savvy dentists will get creative. They will create new rallying points for their community. Here is one cool community project that can be implemented by a dental office without the need to bring people physically together. Your practice can sponsor a digital project for students in the community, build a Facebook following around the project and have parents and other members of the community take part in the project, or do something for the nurses at the local hospital

Or you can swipe and deploy pages out of Dr. Paul Etchison's playbook by asking your community to pick and vote for one charity that you'd support.[18] Dr. Etchison and his Rockstar team at Nelson Ridge Family Dental do this every quarter. From the image overleaf, you can see that the community rallies behind this cause big time. By coming up with a creative way to give back to the Will County community in Illinois, Dr. Paul Etchison and his team have created a great experience that brings the community together.

The key is to pick a cause or target that is easy to get your community to support and be part of. The opportunities are limitless. Imagine how your patients will feel should a project they are part of be featured on TV? Imagine how proud your community will be of both you and itself for having done something great. Imagine how grateful your patients will feel for having you as part of their community.

Fig 18: Nelson Ridge Dental Giving Back

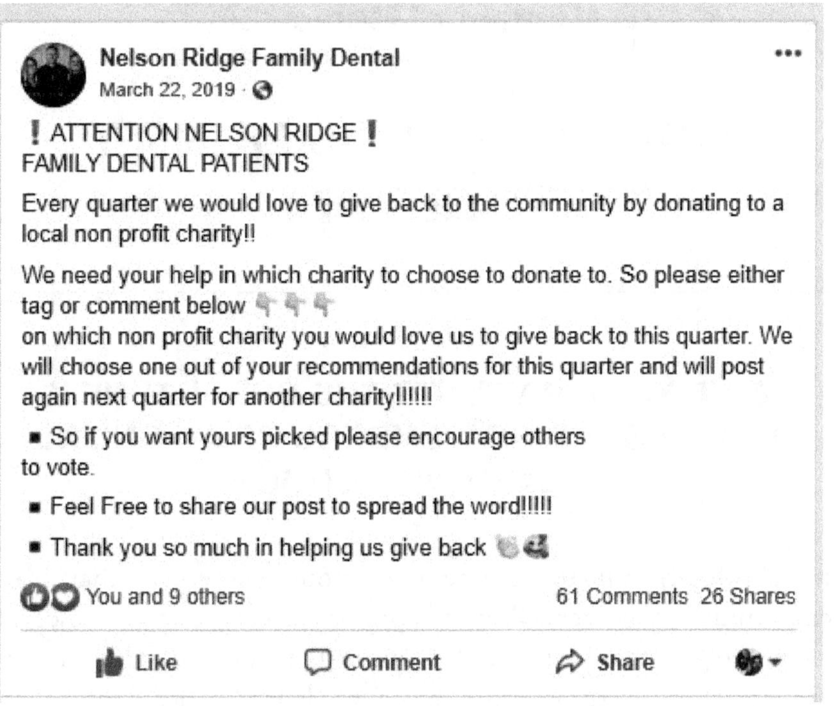

A post on Nelson Ridge Family Dental's Facebook page announcing their quarterly giving back event. This is an awesome way to give back while engaging your community.

BRING THE COMMUNITY TOGETHER

GIVE YOUR PATIENTS THE OPPORTUNITY TO BE FOUNDING MEMBERS OF AN ONLINE COMMUNITY GROUP

It's absolutely fair to assume that group gatherings that bring communities together will be a thing of the past for the foreseeable future, all no thanks to the Coronavirus pandemic. This presents some great opportunities for the savvy dentist to lead the way in creating online community platforms where he or she can invite patients and other members of the community to be part of.

Any business that presents an idea like this in the community it operates will be surprised by the enthusiasm people will display. People will appreciate the opportunity to become founding members of a platform that allows them to congregate as a community at a time when traditional methods of getting together in groups have became unsafe — and in some cases, illegal.

All you need to do is start a community Facebook group and bring your team on board to work on building the membership of the group. If you work with a marketing agency that looks after your Social Media like we do, you could have this group starting to grow in a week or two. It is initiatives like these that will give you great reason to write or text your patient base without selling dentistry. Something that makes them look forward to getting emails, voice mail drops, or text messages from you.

There are many people sitting at home waiting for somebody to invite them to be part of something amazing. Imagine your practice leading the conversation on issues that matter to your community.

CELEBRATE AND PROMOTE YOUR PATIENTS

TURN YOUR PATIENTS INTO COMMUNITY CELEBRITIES BY PROMOTING THEM

Average dental businesses spend a lot of time, money, and effort in promoting themselves. Which is great. But yours is not an average practice. If it is, I'm sure you don't want to remain average because in the unforgiving post COVID-19 economy, average dental practices struggle, and their owners, staff ,and families suffer.

So instead of just promoting yourself and your practice, why not build loyalty and inspire positive behavior from your patients by promoting them or their businesses along with your own? Here is how you get this done.

Include non-dentistry related patient profiles on your website, social media pages, and feature patients in your Patient Newsletter. For example, if one of your patients volunteers at the local SPCA, make that one of your monthly patient profiles and promote that on social media, website, and newsletter if you have one. And you should.

If one of your patients has a child doing a special project with say, the Air Cadets, Girl Guides, or something like that, make that a feature on your website's monthly Community Heroes section and promote that on your social media.

Small gestures like these go an exceptionally long way in demonstrating to your community that you care. I know you know what happens when people in your community believe you care. They talk about you; they come to you and they see you as a leader in their community, things that all translate to a fat collections bag at the end of your production month.

People like to share things that make them look good in the eyes of others. So, you can be guaranteed that your community's relationship with your practice will grow deeper when you promote members of that community and support worthy causes in or outside the community.

GIFT THEM BOOKS THEY LOVE

MAKE YOUR PATIENTS FEEL AND KNOW THAT YOU THINK ABOUT WHAT THEY LOVE OR CARE FOR…

The point behind delivering moments of magic is that those moments stringed together give an experience that fulfils your patients, makes them blissful, or said in cruder language, gives them an emotional orgasm. Having a system that captures patients' unique likes, dislikes, and hobbies is central to helping you deliver these unforgettable experiences.

Suppose you know that a business owner patient of yours who is coming in for her scheduled appointment a week from today is a huge Dan Kennedy fan. Actually, this patient confessed to you that she has graduated from being a Dan Kennedy fan to becoming a full-blown disciple.

Armed with this information, you go onto Amazon and buy one of Dan Kennedy's books and have it delivered to you before the patient's scheduled appointment. When the book gets delivered, you write a really thoughtful message, date and sign the book. (Don't forget your practice name though) You then get the book wrapped in nice gift wrap.

When the patient comes for her appointment, you do everything that needs to be done clinically and customer service wise. Then just as you're about to leave the room, you say;

"Oh Angel, before I forget, I got you a little something as a token of thanks for being a wonderful client of ours. Please open after you leave… and if, that is ONLY if… you like the gift…please don't forget to post a picture on social media."

Now, it might sound as if you gave the gift to get the social media post. That is not totally wrong, but that is certainly not the biggest benefit. The biggest win from this is the moment of magic when the patient opens the gift in her car and sees it's a Dan Kennedy book. She will be flooded with the emotion that comes from knowing somebody cared enough to remember what she cares for. And that somebody is you. She will try to remember how you knew she likes Dan Kennedy, never mind the fact that it was her who mentioned it.

If the patient goes ahead and posts something on social media, that is an added bonus. The real win is the solidification of your practice's relationship with her this moment of magic has created.

This is the stuff that makes for patients who pay more, stay longer, and refer more high-quality people your way. I can guarantee you everybody around you never does this.

SECTION 5

MAKE THEM FEEL SAFE

REMOVE MAGNETS FOR VIRUSES

REMOVING MAGAZINES AND BROCHURES IN YOUR WAITING LOUNGE WILL EXPONENTIALLY INCREASE YOUR PATIENTS' SENSE OF SAFETY

Did you see how fast the coronavirus spread in the black light experiment that was conducted by Japan's public broadcasting organization in partnership with health experts? When I watched the experiment on the news, it got me thinking about how the way people touch stuff in a restaurant is much the same way they touch and handle magazines and brochures in dental lounges and waiting rooms around the world.

Do you have magazines and brochures for patients to browse through in your office while they wait? If your answer is yes, then please allow me to pose this follow up question. Do you want to increase your patients' sense of safety in your office? If your answer is yes – which it should be, because you care about your patients and your bottom line – then remove all magazines and brochure holders in your office.

Like most things people put their hands on in the black light experiment, magazines and brochures will safely house germs and viruses waiting for your patients to pick them up.

And you know what you and your staff should do after getting rid of all the magazines and brochures? You should let your patients know that magazines and brochures have been taken out of the office as a safety measure. How do you let the patients know? You have all team members create opportunities to talk about this with patients, you post it on social media and send emails to your patient base.

BE A CLEAN FREAK

DELIVER AN UNCOMPROMISING LEVEL OF CLEANLINESS

Remember one of the goals for having a laser focus on delivering world-class customer service is to attract people with a taste for quality. These are people who want the best things in life and are willing and able to pay top dollar to get them.

One of the best ways to attract this kind of patient is to have uncompromising levels of cleanliness in your practice. At a time when people are super sensitive about hygiene, the last thing you want is to have your patients think your level of cleanliness is average, or God forbid, below average.

Gone are the days when your practice was only cleaned up at the end of the day after the office was closed. Now you want your patients to see your staff wiping operatory chairs after use. You want patients to see your staff wiping waiting lounge seats.

Washrooms/toilets have to be spotless. This means having to make inspections of these facilities on a regular basis to ensure they are clean. Maintaining an inspection log that anybody who uses the washroom can see is a great way to demonstrate your uncompromising attitude towards running a clean practice.

Imagine how a patient feels when they visit your washroom and they see a cleaning or inspection log hanging on the wall showing an inspection every 2 hours.

Is this excessive or over the top? You bet it is. But will it give your patients a feeling of comfort? Absolutely! And that is exactly what you want. To have patients who are comfortable being in your office.

THE CAR WAITING ROOM

HAVE A FULL LOUNGE OF PEOPLE WAITING IN THEIR OWN CARS

There are good chances that social distancing protocols will stay in place for a very long time to come. As people get used to social distancing, patients will not be comfortable walking into a dental office with three or more people sitting in the waiting lounge.

I know this for sure because my 10-year-old daughter refused to sit in the waiting lounge when I took her to see our family doctor after we got in and found four other people sitting there. We had to wait in the car and only got in after one person had left. But that was after we had an argument with another family that was waiting in their car and had made an attempt to get in before us. I'm sure we got there before them, but that's a story for another day.

So, how do you make your patients' waiting experience more comfortable at a time when social distancing has become the new normal? You do what busy restaurants and pharmacies do. You invest in a patient-paging system. Or if you don't want to invest in a full blown busy-restaurant type paging system, you just use a regular phone notification system.

So, when a patient checks in, they are given a paging disk and told to go and wait for their turn in their car. Or they are told to wait in their vehicle and will receive a phone call when it's their turn to see the doctor.

At a busy restaurant, when a table becomes available, the patron's paging disk buzzes. This informs them that their table is ready. So, when Mrs. Jones' turn to be seen comes, her buzzer is activated, or she gets a phone call and she is taken straight to her treatment room without having to wait in the waiting lounge.

Now, that would be a waiting experience to my liking because I know that my chances of spreading whatever germs or virus I have are lowered and the chances of me getting some bug while sitting with three or four other people are also lowered. This is an extremely simple strategy to implement and it tells your patients that you care for their wellbeing.

NO MORE OPENING DOORS

UPGRADE YOUR MANUAL DOORS TO AUTOMATIC DOORS TO MAKE YOUR PATIENTS FEEL SAFER

The last thing patients want bothering their minds is the thought of whether or not they caught a virus of one kind or another while at the dentist. In the same vein, the last thing you and your team wants is to always be bothered by the thought of some devil of a virus hanging around your practice door handle. Doors are a special magnet for germs because everybody touches them to go in and out of rooms and the practice itself.

So how do you put your patients at ease and make them feel comfortable as they come or leave your office? Easy, but this costs a bit. Sooner or later, dentists that want to remove people's fears and increase people's confidence will have to do this. So, what is this?

It's the installation of automatic doors. Automatic doors in and out of your practice ensure that people don't bring germs by touching the doors. And when you have the automatic doors installed, talk about it on social media to let your patients know when they come in. The bottom line is to make a big deal out of this, so that your patients can see the lengths you're going to ensure their safety and peace of mind.

Moment of Magic #41

GIVE AN OFFICE TOUR LIKE NO OTHER

GIVE A SAFE OFFICE TOUR EXPERIENCE IN THE AGE OF COVID BY DEPLOYING AN IMMERSIVE DIGITAL TOUR, NOT A PHYSICAL TOUR[19]

For the business savvy dentist who is hell bent on creating the ultimate new patient experience, the days of taking their new patients on a physical tour of the office are long gone. According to Dr. Dustin Burleson, who runs the 8-figure Burleson Orthodontics, the physical office tour has several disadvantages.

For starters, it's difficult to control the new patient experience when the patient is taken around various parts of the practice. The chances of having a new patient have a negative experience by for example, seeing a patient having a tooth pulled out or somebody throwing up, are high. To add to the possibility of a new patient having a negative experience, it's impossible to re-create the same experience every time a new patient is taken on a physical tour.

So how do you deliver an experience that wows every new patient each time the office tour is given? You create a digital office tour, as opposed to having a physical tour. According to Dr. Burleson, the most critical part of designing your digital office tour is to ensure it showcases every element of your practice in terms of the benefits that element has for the patient. Focus on the direct benefits to the patient.

To create a digital office tour that gives your patient a remarkable experience, you must script the digital tour and have professional photos and videos taken. When you have all the elements in place, you must have a professional video editor put all the elements together into one emotionally-charged presentation that builds up and credentializes you as the dentist, showcases the community work you do, and showcases your high tech equipment in terms of the benefits to the patient. Have the presentation highlight what makes your practice unique, showcase stories of transformation by other patients, show fun office activities your staff undertakes as well as your own family, staff and their families.

The main goal with your digital tour is to demonstrate to the new patient that by choosing your office, they are choosing a practice that cares and that makes a difference in their community.

Besides presenting you with the golden opportunity to deliver the emotional experience that makes it easiest for your new patients to like and trust you, the digital tour also helps lower the risk of spreading the Corona virus by limiting the number of people walking around the practice.

Dr. Burleson swears by the digital office tour's power to deliver the kind of experience that makes for strong bonds being created between your practice and its new patients. So, while the average dentist struggles to figure out how to safely showcase their practice to new patients, the business savvy dentist deploys a well-crafted, emotionally charged digital tour that builds and solidifies their relationship with new patients from day one.

SECTION 6

THE 9-STAR FOLLOW UP

DON'T ACT LIKE YOU ONLY CARE FOR THEIR MONEY

DEMONSTRATE THAT YOU CARE AND ARE GRATEFUL BY NOT ONLY SHOWING UP IN YOUR PATIENTS' INBOXES IN THE FORM OF A PAYMENT RECEIPT

Our two girls' teeth are really messed up. I'm convinced those chewing organs have a mind of their own. They just come up wherever they feel like coming up, on top of each other, beside each other and get this – some that should have fallen out when it was time to go decided to stay in place a wee bit longer, forcing the new teeth to take matters into their own hands and just come out anyway. So, to say my girls' mouths are a mess is an understatement. Which is why we went out in search of an orthodontist.

The wife did her due diligence and we checked out two offices close to our home. We finally settled on one based on their excellent payment plan, the friendliness of the staff and the overall feel of the office. Victoria's case was pretty straight forward; so within a few weeks, she had her braces slapped. Angel's case was a little more complicated; so she needed more x-rays done, then Covid happened. She still has to have her treatment started but like I said, Victoria's treatment is already underway starting March. I'm writing this towards the end of May. That's three months in.

Within these last three months would you guess how many times the orthodontic office that will be getting about $7500 from me has written to me or my wife? Three times. And can you guess what the three communications were? Payment receipts.

Yes, I need to get the payment receipts each time a payment goes through. But what does sending me receipts as the **only** message I get tell me about my orthodontist? I don't know about you, but as far as I'm concerned, this tells me this orthodontist doesn't care about my kids' teeth at all. The husband and wife team are only interested in getting my money. If I could, I would most certainly cancel the treatment and find somebody that cares.

How about sending a simple text (which can be easily automated) asking after how my kid is doing? How has she adjusted to having braces in her mouth? How about sending us some resources to help her maintain the braces? Is this not how to demonstrate you care as opposed to just sending me receipts?

I like what Dr. Craig Spodak over at Spodak Dental once said when he pointed out that the ultimate purpose of a business is to provide compassion, trust, and love.[20] For practices that don't care for their patients, the provision of compassion, trust and love stops right after the patient has signed the contract.

If your goal is demonstrating that you care and not have somebody who gets annoyed each time they get your payment receipt, then don't do what my kids' orthodontist is doing. It doesn't take much to have an automated system send messages asking after the progress and health of a patient.

Fig 19: Demonstrating You Care...Like Friend

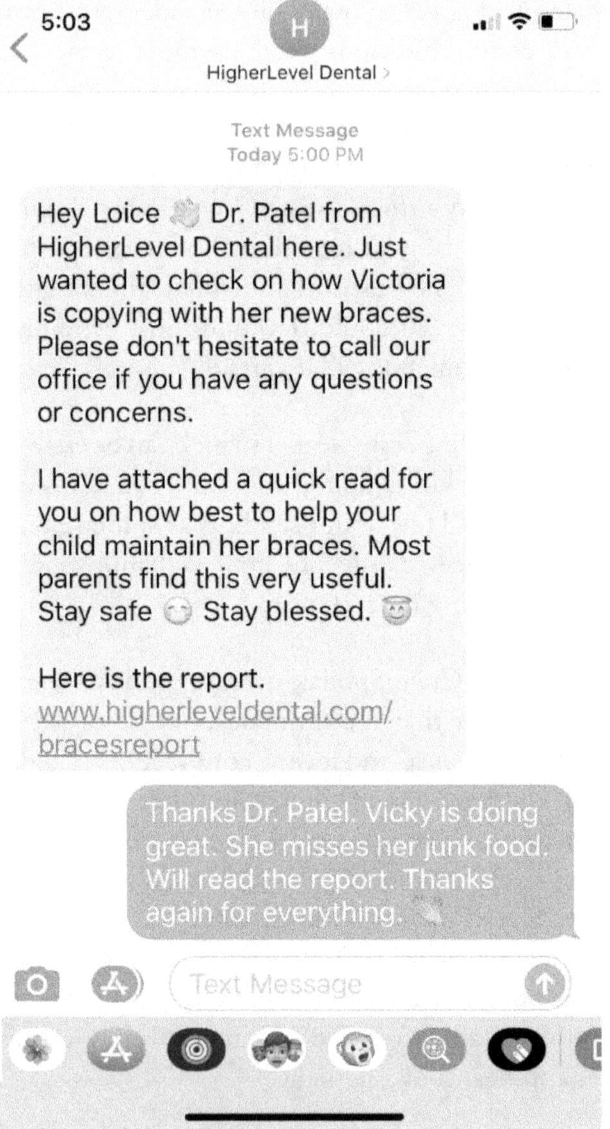

CONTINUE CARING EVEN WHEN THEY STOP COMING

MAKE INACTIVE PATIENTS APPRECIATE YOU CONTINUING TO CARE ABOUT THEM, EVEN WHEN THEY STOPPED COMING TO SEE YOU

How would you feel if you were to receive a handwritten letter, a text message, and then a phone call from a friend you haven't seen in a long time? Let's say you decide to put your friend to the test, and you don't respond to any of the messages. How will you feel, or what will you think were your friend to continue sending messages using various channels? If you're like most people, you'd be convinced that your friend cares a lot. If you had gone your separate ways on bad terms, you would be convinced of their genuine desire to make amends

As a dental practice owner, you have patients who haven't come back to see you in a long time. You call these 'friends', your inactive patients. Most of them would appreciate it very much were they to hear from you offering them something to do with dentistry or you just wanting to ask after their health and life. There are businesses that I have switched away from that I would seriously consider going back to patronize if I should get a message from them just reaching out and inviting me to come back.

Who doesn't want to be told that they are missed? If you put in place a system to predictably reach out to your base of inactive patients, you'd be surprised how the one time work of setting up the system will bring in a consistent flow of patients who would otherwise be dormant. Why? Because people are always open to rekindling relationships after being told they are missed.

So, what does your inactive patient reactivation system look like? Is it bringing you a consistent flow of patients that would otherwise have remained inactive had you not reached out to them?

If you believe that your inactive patient reactivation needs a serious make over, please get in touch. We'll be more than happy to show you what you can do to supercharge your patient reactivation. Long lost friends are always happy to hear from their colleagues when a good message comes in just to check on them.

Fig 20: Patient Reactivation Postcard Sample[21]

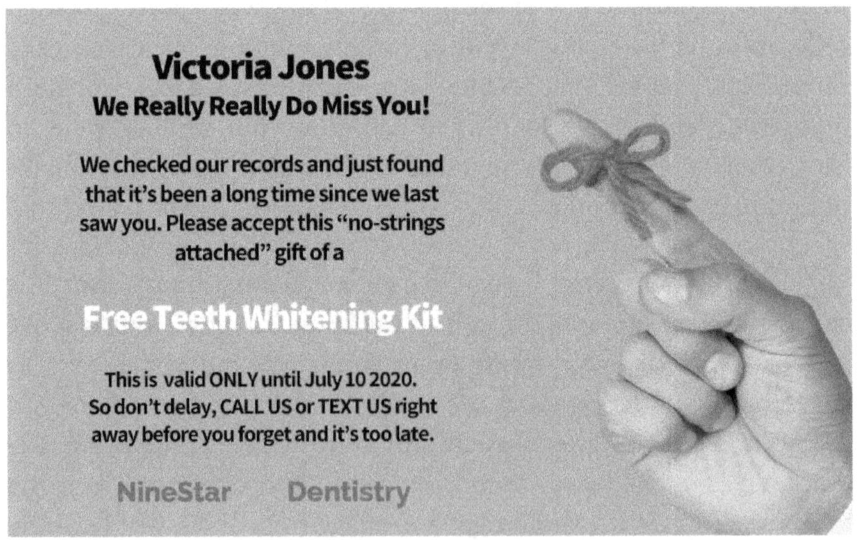

Fig 21: Patient Reactivation Text Message

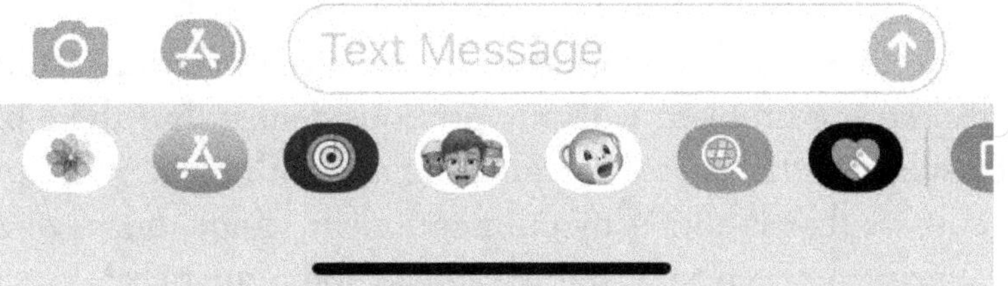

DON'T ANNOY PATIENTS WITH IRRELEVANT MESSAGES

Imagine how annoyed 30-year-old Janice would get when she receives a text message offering her 40% discount on dentures from her dentist. Or how 65-year-old Mrs. James feels when she gets an email or flyer for Invisalign. The very last thing you want to do is annoy your patients for no reason. Not saying that there is any valid reason for annoying your patients, but you get what I'm saying.

The point is this, when it comes to your automated follow-up, you want your patients to experience the same world-class customer service just as if they were sitting in your office. There is no point in sending emails or text messages about implants or dentures to a mom who's had braces for her kids. Why not follow up to check on how the kids are adjusting to life with braces? How about following up to check if the kids or family is having any issues?

The other day, I discussed the possibility of getting a solution for my snoring problem with my previous dentist, but there in my inbox was an offer for teeth-whitening a month later. What in the heavens was that about? Why unintentionally annoy the very people whose help you need to guarantee you a good retirement?

The solution to not annoying your patients with communication that is irrelevant to them lies in personalizing the follow up messages to the exact treatment that you have given. You do this by segmenting your patients according to the treatments they have received, or the treatment options you have already discussed with them.

This is where a good marketing automation tool comes in handy. You want one that enables you to pinpoint with laser-targeted accuracy which of your patients got what treatment and then deploy marketing messages that are customized for just those patients. And you want the messages to be providing value more than it sells procedures.

Fig 22: Marketing Automation Dashboard

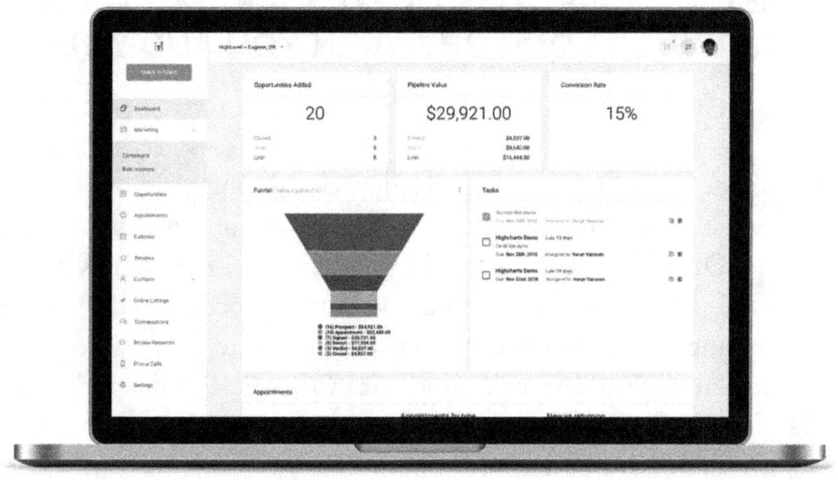

Use cutting edge marketing automation to send targeted messages that are relevant to your patients. Imagine how annoying it is to receive an email that welcomes you back for an appointment when all you did was sign up to receive a newsletter on a dental website.

SURPRISE THEM WITH A POST-OP CALL OR TEXT

HOW MAKING A FOLLOW UP PHONE CALL TO CHECK ON A PATIENT AFTER A PROCEDURE CREATES A BOND BETWEEN YOU AND YOUR PATIENTS

One of the reasons people cancel dental appointments or do not go to see a dentist is the all too common fear of dentistry among humans. One of the reasons for this fear is pain. I don't know about you, but I don't like pain – and a few dental procedures do involve pain ranging from moderate to extreme. How one defines moderate and extreme depends on one's tolerance for pain. For me and many other people, all pain has just but one range. 10 – 10.

So, knowing that humans have a hate-hate relationship with pain, and knowing that with some dental procedures, pain is unavoidable, you have an excellent opportunity to give a 9-Star Experience to a patient who has just gone through a pain or discomfort-inducing procedure. Here is how to create the moment of magic.

Exactly 24 hours after the pain inducing procedure has been performed, drop the patient a quick phone voice mail to check on them. And you don't have to take time out of your day to send this message. Have the voice mail message send as part of your post procedure automated Follow-Up Campaign.

If you're an above average dentist, you send this voice mail message and leave it at that. But if you're a business savvy, way above average dentist, you'll go one step further.

You'd send, say 10 minutes after the voice mail drop, a quick voice mail message like the one on the next page. Now that is what I call going over and above the call of duty to wow the patient by demonstrating that you care. Patients who get this level of attention and care will reciprocate by going out their way to stay with you and refer every breathing human within their circle of influence.

Fig 23: Sample Dentist Follow Up Text

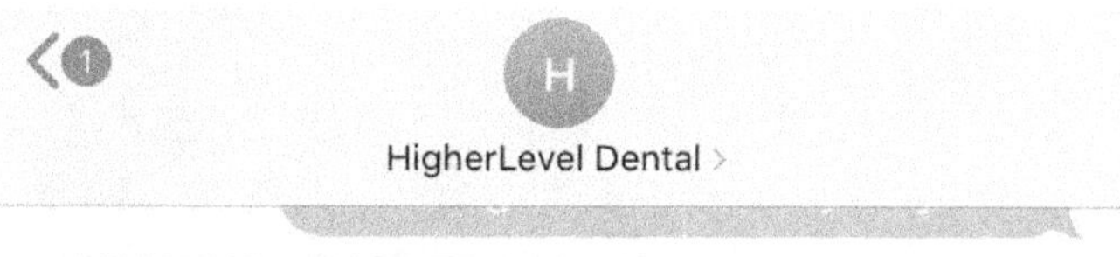

SECTION 7

THE 9-STAR TEAM EXPERIENCE

Fig 24: Focusing On The Wrong Things?

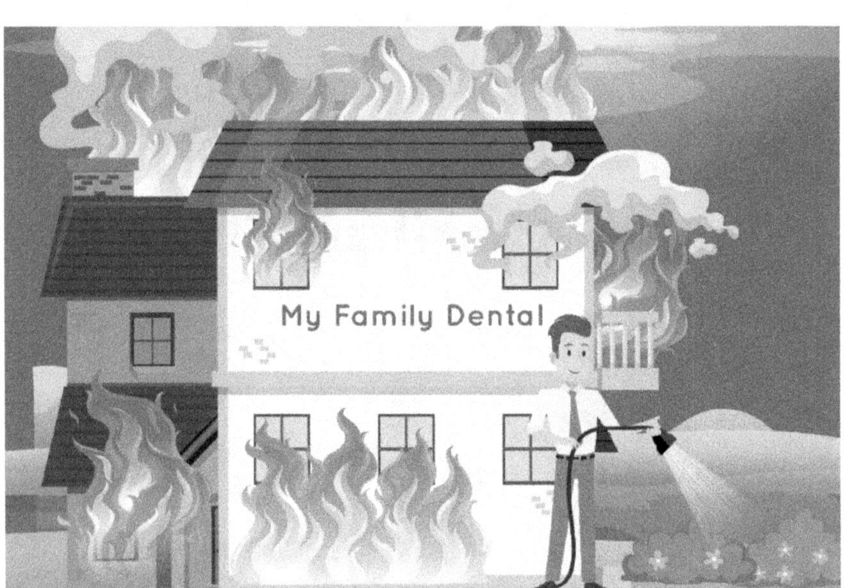

Your TEAM Is Your Practice... Focusing On Much Else
Before A 9-Star Team Experience Is Attained Is Like Aiming
A Fire Hose On Flowers When Your House Is Burning.

THE 9-STAR TEAM EXPERIENCE

GIVING YOUR STAFF THE 9-STAR EXPERIENCE IS THE BEST THING YOU CAN DO TO CREATE A WORK CULTURE THAT WILL GUARANTEE A SECURE FINANCIAL FUTURE FOR YOU, YOUR STAFF, YOUR FAMILY, AND THEIR FAMILIES

According to the amazing Dr. Paul Etchison over at Nelson Ridge Family Dental in New Lenox, Illinois, having an amazing Team Experience is the master key to your patients getting the 9-Star Experience upon which your growth depends.

Every successful leader in dentistry from Dr. Howard Farran[22] to Dr. Rinesh Ganatra agrees.[23] Having built a team of 100 front desk, concierge, valet, and protection services staff serving some of Toronto's upscale high-rise condominiums, I know a thing or two about doing what it takes to create a team experience that makes staff members identify with the mission and go all out in support of its execution.

This section will be providing you with gems you can use starting today to give your staff a Team Experience that will have them running over themselves to please the patients. This is about simple strategies you can deploy to create a great culture for your practice – with the end goal being to have a team that excels in delivering the 9-Star Patient Experience every time.

Moment of Magic #47

A FUN-FILLED OFFICE DOESN'T SUCK TO COME TO

THE POWER OF CREATING A FUN WORKING ENVIRONMENT AND CULTURE

Have you ever visited or moved to a new team and found yourself in the midst of an environment where fun doesn't exist? If you have, which is highly likely, then you know how hard it is, for the camaraderie needed to excel, to exist. This is especially evident in business environments where people whose work and success at that work depends on each other much more closely – environments like dental and orthodontic offices.

The fun element of a dental or orthodontic office is an integral part of the practice's personality. We all love to be around people with great personalities. Being around them is such a great experience that, if possible, one would love to repeat many times. The same with every dental practice, it has a personality. So, what is the personality of your practice? If your office was a person, which person you know would it be?

The other day I was listening to the Dental Heroes podcast and Dr. Etchison stressed the importance of having an intentional strategy to make your practice a happy and fun place. Fred Joyal, in his book, *Becoming Remarkable,* went to great lengths discussing why it's crucial for the dentist and his team to make an extra effort to make the practice a great place to work.[24]

Like the experience of being around someone with a great personality, your patients will enjoy the experience of coming into your office for treatment. The fun and inviting personality of your office culture will go a long way in dissolving the perennial fear of coming to the dentist that most living humans are cursed with.

You and your leadership team must work hard to 'police' your culture against toxic members of the team. How happy your team is, is the most important determinant of whether or not your patients enjoy a great experience – which is the best thing for your production and collections.

A TEAM THAT READS TOGETHER LEADS THE PACK

START AND PROMOTE THE READING CULTURE IN YOUR PRACTICE

I'm sure you've heard the saying, *leaders are readers.* It is true because all leaders are readers in real life. You know this. I'm sure you also know that most successful teams read and practice a lot to hone their craft as a team. Do you have a defined strategy for getting your team to become a reading team? Is everyone on the same page when it comes to what is expected of them and their team-mates as far as delivering superior customer service is concerned?

All the great pro sports coaches from Phil Jackson to Bill Belichick are known for having made it mandatory for their players to read certain prescribed books. This practice made sure everybody was on the same page when it came to strategies, plays and mindset.

Just communicating the importance of reading the same books as a team does wonders in giving them a great sense of belonging and building the desire to pull forward in giving patients an experience of a lifetime. In this day and age, getting people to develop and improve themselves using books is easier than it has ever been. Those in your team who like to read actual hard copies can do so; those who prefer listening can do so, and those who like to use their digital devices can also do so.

To begin this culture in your practice, you, as the leader must buy copies of a great book for each of your team members. Get audio versions for those who prefer listening, Kindle versions for those who prefer Kindle, and hard copies for those who love the feel of pages on their hands. To derive the greatest benefit from this, you must make the reading of these books a mandatory requirement for your staff.

And you must agree with your team on deadlines by which each book must be finished so that everybody is on the same page when it comes time to discussing the lessons and choosing what strategies to implement. Will you get pushback from some members of your team? Possibly. But as long as you communicate the vision and goals you have for doing this and have them be involved in the selection of books to read, those against the idea will come around.

When I was working to take my company's delivery of upscale concierge services to the next level, what I described above is exactly what I did. I gave my teams copies of Tony Hsieh's *Delivering Happiness*, Isadore *Sharp's Four Seasons: The Story of A Business Philosophy*, as well as multiple books on Nordstrom. The teams at our various upscale properties knew that reading the books within the agreed time frames was non-negotiable, if they wanted to keep their well-paying jobs that came with full benefits.

Here is a small challenge for you to get started. Get David Goggins' book, *Can't Hurt Me: Master Your Mind and Defy The Odds*. Just get it for two or three members of your team and have them read or listen to it with their loved ones. Just watch what happens after they read or listen to the book. It's amazing. The mindset shift in your people will shock you.

Moment of Magic #49

USE FBI TYPE INTEL ON YOUR STAFF

BUILD A SECRET SERVICE FILE OF INTELLIGENCE ON YOUR TEAM

Dr. David Moffet, author of the highly instructional bestseller, *How To Build The Dental Practice Of Your Dreams: (Without Killing Yourself!) In Less Than 60 Days,* teaches on the importance of you and your staff developing a secret service mindset for use in collecting intelligence about your patients. Intelligence that will be useful in future interactions with the patients as a way of demonstrating that you care.

I would like to propose that you, the owner of your practice, along with your team leader(s) develop your own secret service information repository on your staff.

Yeah, I know. It does sound like you will be spying on your staff. But no, you will not be spying on your staff. What you will do is create a system that gets your staff to volunteer personal information on themselves. Information on things like their hobbies, names of children, things their loved ones enjoy, their dreams, aspirations, and significant events in their lives. Make this information repository dynamic, so that that new information is always being added and updated and old information taken out.

One of the best things you can do is give everybody access to this information. This makes it easier for the team to give into each other, all contributing to creating an awesome Team Experience. Now, when you have the file of information on your staff, it's time to start using that information to create moments of magic for your team. The very act of having your team all together to create this information repository is a great culture-building exercise. Encourage every member of the team to take the initiative in creating moments of magic amongst each other.

Imagine how your culture will evolve when all your staff members go out of their way to surprise each other with gifts on special occasions and family anniversaries, with offers of help, or by supporting each other in unique ways based on the information in the secret information repository.

One of the best ways to get a deeper appreciation of your team's aspirations is having each member create and share a vision board. Knowing your team members' deepest aspirations, gives them a sense that you care for them. It also helps you know with absolute certainty what goals to help them achieve. This strategy has been responsible for Dr. Glenn Vo's success.[25]

LOVE ON YOUR TEAM'S LOVED ONES

SHOW THAT YOU REALLY CARE FOR YOUR TEAM'S LOVED ONES.

Everyone on your team belongs to a family. One of the best ways you can create an awesome experience for your team is to demonstrate that you, the CEO of your practice, care for their family members. Former President Obama and former Prime Minister of Canada, Jean Chretien are famous for shocking their staff with their knowledge of the staff members' private lives. President Obama went the furthest distance in this regard by going as far as buying presents during important dates in the lives of people close to his members of staff.

Imagine how a junior staffer felt when out of the blue, a senior staffer handed her a birthday present for her mom from the President. How on earth did he remember, is all that came to the junior staffer's mind as emotions overcame her with love for her President. Imagine the lengths this staffer would from then on be willing to go in support of President Obama's initiatives. Your staff will feel and do the same to help your mission to deliver the most outstanding patient experience if you go out of your way to show them that you care for the people they love.

This is where having a deep reservoir of tidbits of knowledge about your staff comes handy. The more information you have at your disposal, the more creative you can get, and the sky is the limit. Imagine at the end of the year how your team culture would have developed when in the last 12 months, every member of your team had someone they love receive a gift or present of some sort from the practice team? Imagine the stories around the office? Is that not fodder for outrageous referrals growth coming right from your team? And the team camaraderie! That will just go through the roof.

FRESHEN UP YOUR TEAM'S LOOK

GIVE YOUR PATIENTS A TEAM THAT SHOWS UP IN STYLISH AND FRESH WORK ATTIRE THAT IS WELCOMING AND HAS A PERSONALITY...EVEN IF THE ATTIRE HAS TO BE COVERED BY PPE

One of the things that hit you when you enter the orbit of any service delivered on the Ritz-Carlton Yacht, Residency or Hotel is the dressing of the staff – The Ladies and Gentlemen who serve Ladies and Gentlemen. They are dressed to deliver the presence of an upscale experience.

If you've not been to a Ritz-Carlton or Four Seasons, just do a simple search online for how their staff looks. Now compare that to the work attire your staff uses. Most dental practices still hang on to the idea of having their staff look like hospital staff. While it's absolutely correct that you are operating a medical services business, having members of your staff dressed like hospital staff will result in your practice getting slaughtered in the new economy.

Dentists who will thrive in the new economy understand this one fact – that to thrive, they MUST deploy a well-designed customer service experience. And doing that demands having their staff show up and present that experience dressed like service rockstars.

Yes, even with all the COVID-19 PPE requirements, your staff have to show up dressed to impress.

So, how does your staff's scrubs game look like right now? Ask them what they think. If the funds are there, make the investment in upscale scrubs for your team. Make them look great, the effect will add to giving your patients a 9-Star Experience along with the accompanying boosts in production.

BUILD A TEAM OF FBI AGENTS

HAVE YOUR TEAM COLLECT INTELLIGENCE ON PATIENTS LIKE FBI AGENTS...OR THE EQUIVALENT

Foundational to delivering the 9-Star Experience is your team's ability to make patients feel and know that whoever they interact with actually listens to them, is genuinely interested and cares for them. According to a report by Small Business Trends, 68% of customers leave because they perceive the service providers to be indifferent. I know this firsthand with the experience I had with my last dental office and I know you know this too.

So how do you and your team demonstrate that you genuinely care and are interested in your patients? First everybody in your practice must develop the mentality of an FBI agent – or whatever your nation's top investigations agency is called. They must use every interaction with the patient to gather useful information and then deploy this information in future communications and interactions with the patients.

Suppose Fatima, your hygienist, used her FBI agent intelligence-collecting skills the last time Mrs. Andrews came in and found out that her son was getting married in a week. Fatima had the front desk team record this vital piece of information in Mrs. Andrews' file. When the front desk team was going through the next day's appointments, they took notice of the fact that Mrs. Andrews was coming in, so they brought this fact to your attention as well as that of the dental assistant.

As the dentist hell bent on creating awesome experiences for your patients, you have a nice congratulations card done and a gift card placed in the card for the newlyweds. You get everybody on the team to sign the card.

Now imagine how Mrs. Andrews is going to feel when she gets the gift for her son and daughter-in-law from you and your team. Imagine what goes through her mind when you, Fatima or another member of your team inquires with unbridled enthusiasm how her son's wedding went? Imagine also what the son and daughter-in-law will think when they get the wedding gift from mom's dentist?

Many good things are going to happen for your practice as a result of deploying this strategy. Mrs. Andrews will know you and your team care not just for her, but for the people she loves as well. Her trust in you and your team will go through the roof and she will not stop talking about you and your team whenever an opportunity to do so comes up.

Now, you have many friends in the dental profession, who do you know who has done this? Chances are high that you would be hard pressed to find any dentist who goes to these sorts of lengths to create these kinds of out-of-body experiences for their patients. Is this over the top? You bet it is over the top, but Doc, you're building your practice in the post Covid-19 era. In order to attract high value clients, you're going to have to provide over the top customer service experiences for your patients. If you don't, whichever dentist does will take all your clients away.

SECTION 8

THE 9-STAR PATIENT EXPERIENCE

DITCH THE PAPER AND CLIP BOARD

MAKE IT SUPER EASY AND SAFE FOR NEW PATIENTS TO PROVIDE YOU WITH THE INFORMATION YOU NEED TO TREAT AND WOW THEM

Isn't it crazy that even with the Coronavirus pandemic, there are some medical facilities that still use paper forms and clip boards to capture patient information?

And when a terrified patient asks if there was another way to provide their information that does not involve touching an item that is a magnet for germs and viruses, they are told they can do it on the website on a computer – at home, because the facility won't have devices where patients can't log in to provide their information. This is so 2019 and it will drive patients away.

Making patients feel safe by doing away with the paper registration forms and the clipboard must be a no brainer in the post-Coronavirus world. The savvy Dentist will have a tablet for use by walk-in new patients to register themselves as well as have his or her registration forms available on the practice website for filling up there without the need for having to print them.

Anything that will make people feel safe is a great experience in the current environment and in the future. Invest in digital tablets and ditch the clipboard. Your patients will appreciate it very much. My dentist has done this, and I am truly appreciative.

Fig 25: Go Digital With Patient Information Collection

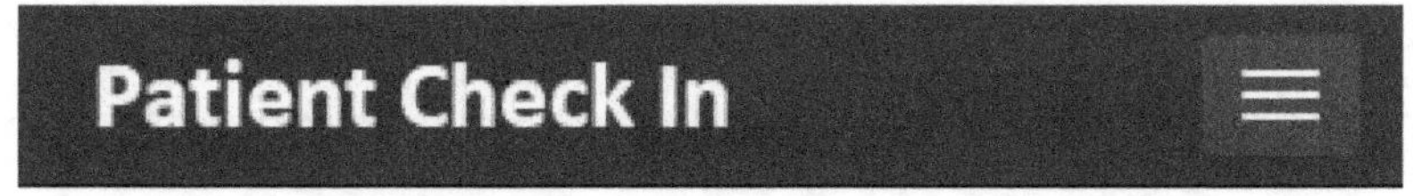

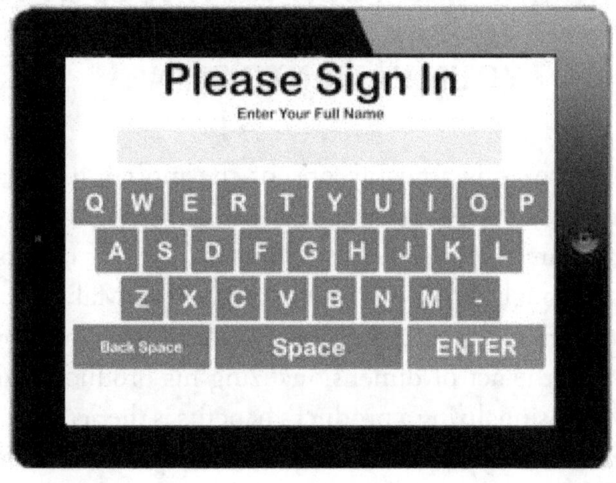

Moment of Magic #54

MAKE YOUR EQUIPMENT BENEFITS SIZZLE

DIMENSIONALIZE YOUR TECHNOLOGY AND EQUIPMENT TO MAKE ITS DIRECT BENEFITS TO YOUR PATIENTS SHINE

Clayton Makepeace is arguably one of the most influential direct response copywriters who's ever lived. He deployed copywriting strategies that are responsible for selling millions of dollars' worth of products through direct mail. One of Clayton Makepeace's most effective strategies that created a magnetic emotional appeal for his products is the act of dimensionalizing his products' functional benefits. Dimensionalizing a product's benefits is the act of presenting those benefits as they apply to the problems, pains, and challenges faced by the consumer of the product. [26]

How does all this apply to you and your desire to deliver a patient experience that'll exponentially increase your case acceptance and practice growth? Well, the way you and your team present technology to your patients always does one of two things depending on how the presentation is done.

The presentation experience either leaves the patient with no clear understanding of how the technology applies to him/her, or it leaves the patient fully appreciating the technology as a result of having a deep understanding of what the technology means to his or her problems. To have his patients leave the office and go evangelize about his technology to friends and loved ones, the savvy Dentist will communicate his technology's benefits as they apply to his patients. In other words, the savvy Dentist will dimensionalize the benefits of his or her equipment so that the patients clearly see how they get to benefit.

In real terms, this means presenting for example, cone beam technology in terms of its ability to save patients' time, allowing them faster recovery and drastically reducing their fears of radiation exposure.

For your team to consistently deliver the same message on the benefits (as they apply to your patients) of all your equipment and technology, you must train and have them work from documented marketing and customer service delivery SOPs.

Like the amazing Dr. Etchison at Nelson Ridge Family Dental likes to teach, your team must know and understand the rules of the game in order for them to play to win. Clearly documenting how each functional element of your technology benefits the patients is clarifying those rules to win. And in this case, winning is having an increasing case acceptance rate that comes from patients having trust in the equipment and technology you have invested in on their behalf.

Fig 26: Burning Cash Through Advertising?

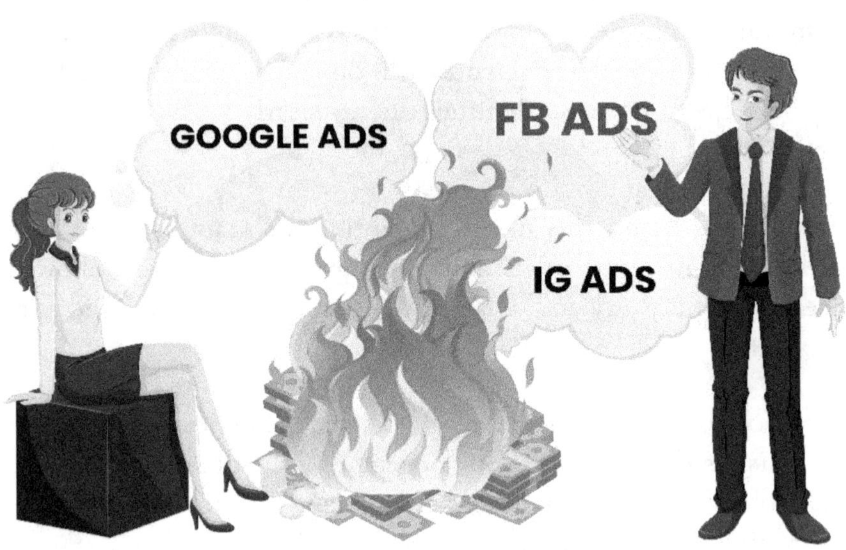

The main reason most dental ads don't bring great results is their failure to make emotional connections that appeal to their intended audience. Have you ever asked yourself what emotional experience the people you intend to act on your ads should have as they consume your advertising? If you haven't asked yourself this question, or if you have, but have not figured out an answer, then you might as well be burning your cash. Get in touch with our team at www.9spe.com/strategy. We'll point you in the right direction.

THE ART OF BUILDING UP THE DENTIST

MAKE YOUR NEW PATIENTS BELIEVE YOU'RE THE BEST DENTIST TO HAVE WALKED THE FACE OF THE EARTH...BEFORE THEY EVEN MEET YOU IN PERSON

How much does your staff build you up as the Dentist during those precious moments before you meet a patient for the very first time? Did you know that according to Dr. Burleson, the act of building up and credentializing the dentist creates the kind of trust that make patients' resistance to treatment melt like butter at the touch of a hot knife?

Remember these are the ultimate goals in all this – to make the new patients as comfortable as possible and to get them to give the dentist their total trust, just as airline travelers totally give their total trust to their pilot.

Based on his extensive experience, both in his own practice and with his consulting clients around the world, Dr. Burleson knows that the staff member who interacts with the patient last, before the dentist meets the patient for the very first time has a huge responsibility – the responsibility of building up the dentist in the eyes of the new patient. Call it, if you will, priming the patient to meet, and be favorably disposed to consider the doctor's recommendations.

The experience of having somebody else talk about the Dentist in glowing - but not exaggerated - terms builds trust in the patient. The kind of trust that drastically reduces the patient's anxiety and makes for a positive treatment or consultation experience.

So how does the Dentist get built up before he or she meets the new patient for the very first time? Again, according to Dr. Burleson, the team member prepping the new patient to meet the dentists for the first time must credentialize and build up the Doctor before the Doctor gets into the operatory.

The assistant talks about the Doctor's life points; what charities he supports, his hobbies, family as well as any other highlights that would make the patient think, *"ummm this Dentist is awesome, I can't wait to meet him."* By building up the doctor in this way, a bond of trust will have started to form between the patient and the dentist before the dentist shows his face, which is exactly what you want to see happening.

The process of credentializing and building up the dentist would have started in the Digital Office Tour, or if you still do physical office tours, it would have started there.

SOLIDIFY THEIR TRUST IN YOU BY USING A SHOCK & AWE PACKAGE

USE A SHOCK & AWE PACKAGE TO GIVE NEW PATIENTS A WELCOME EXPERIENCE THAT CREATES ABSOLUTE TRUST IN YOU

Dan Kennedy is arguably the most influential direct response marketing authority to have walked the face of planet earth. Businesses that have implemented his strategies have experienced 2X, 3X or even 10X growth. One of the strategies that Dan is infamous for is building and deploying a Shock and Awe Package. [27]

The purpose of the Shock & Awe Package is to give your new patients a welcome experience like no other. The contents of the package positively reinforce the patient's decision to choose your practice while at the same time positioning you as the undisputed dental or orthodontic authority in your community.

The average dentist will deploy a new patient package containing a brochure or two, toothbrushes, toothpaste, floss, and lip balm. Nothing more. The savvy dentist who's made it his or her mission to build a practice that will sell for a fat 7 or 8 figure lumpsum will take a leaf out of Dr Dustin Burleson's playbook when it comes to building a new patient package.

Dr Dustin Burleson - Owner of the 8-Figure practice, Burleson Orthodontics, and longtime student of Dan Kennedy – once asked during a webinar; what is the most valuable asset that establishes a dentist's or orthodontist's authority as he or she walks into case presentations. The Shock & Awe Package came up in the top three.

As a dentist or Orthodontist, you want your patients to trust you the way you would trust your pilot if you were boarding a plane. The pilot's authority is beyond question. You literally put your life in his or her hands and trust that everything he or she does or recommends is for your own good. That's exactly how you want patients to see you. Now, how do you establish that kind of authority in your community and target market especially with new people?

Simple. Get your new patients to experience your Shock and Awe Package. To be effective, your Shock and Awe Package needs to be built according to the master's specifications – Dan Kennedy's. The team at The Dentistry Funnel is available to walk you through the building of your Shock and Awe Package. Send us a message and we'll be happy to point you in the right direction. Or better still, we'll be more than happy to work with you to build the package that will give you the same authority on your new patients that an airline pilot has over his or her passengers.

SURPRISE THEM WITH A WELCOME PHONE CALL

DRASTICALLY CUT DOWN THE NUMBER OF NEW PATIENT NO-SHOWS BY SENDING A WELCOME PHONE CALL...ON AUTOPILOT

According to Fred Joyal, one of the co-founders at 1-800-DENTIST, 50% of new patients never return to a dental practice after the first visit. That's some scary statistic if you ask me. Mr. Joyal and his team have spent over half a billion dollars in advertising just for dentists, so the man knows dental patients.

So, if there is a possibility that half of your new patients will not come back after the first visit, what can you do as business savvy dentist to increase the chances of your new patients coming back? You obviously want the number of non-returnees dropping down to zero if possible, but how do you get that done?

One way you can get this done is by demonstrating beyond the shadow of any doubt that you, the dentist, and owner of the practice, genuinely care for every new patient who comes in for a free consultation or treatment. All this is good, but how do you demonstrate that you care for a new patient who has had their first visit?

First of all, I hope it is a cultural norm in your practice that every new patient gets to meet the dentist on their first visit. If not, this is something that needs to be corrected.

So, assuming that the new patient has had the opportunity to meet the dentist, 24 hours after this initial visit a voice mail is dropped saying something along these lines…

"Hey there. Dr. Divine here from HigherLevel Dental. Just wanted to let you know that it was an absolute pleasure meeting you yesterday. The entire team loved your energy and we're looking forward to seeing you again on your next appointment. Stay safe."

You then follow up this voice mail drop 10 minutes later with a text message along the same lines.

The most beautiful thing about these messages is that they can all be automated. You or your team don't have to lift a finger or do anything once they are set. Like the master of infomercials Ronald Popeil used to say when peddling his Showtime Rotisserie on TV – you set it and forget it.

What these messages do is to confirm in the mind of the patient that he or she has made a wise decision choosing you as their dentist. It is this positive conformation that will help in getting all your follow-up messages read – that's assuming you have a good follow-up system in place - and not be thrown into the trash. One of the reasons these messages work to increase the number of new patients who come back is that very few professional service providers do this. So, you doing this will make you stand out head and shoulders above everybody else in the city.

Fig 27: Dentist's New Patient WOW Text

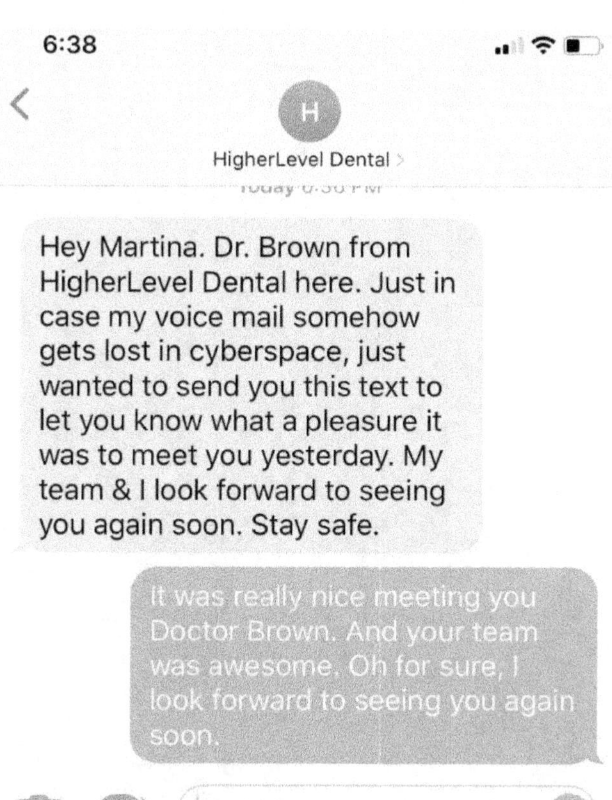

Example of the type of follow up text message to a new patient that will have them looking forward to coming back for their next appointment.

SECTION 8

CASE ACCEPTANCE EXPLODING EXPERIENCE

DON'T BREAK THE THREE RINGS RULE

MAKE THEM FEEL SOMEBODY IS ALWAYS AVAILABLE TO ANSWER THEIR CALLS

I've been watching The Last Dance, the story of Michael Jordan and The Chicago Bulls on Netflix. One of the most important lessons I've taken from the series is the importance of deploying a few key strategies in pursuit of creating a winning Team Experience. One such key strategy for the Bulls was the Triangle Offense Strategy. Under legendary coach Phil Jackson, the Bulls won a whooping six NBA championships playing the Triangle Offence Strategy.

Is there one strategy that if implemented in a dental practice would result in increases in production and collections similar to the Chicago Bulls winnings as a result of the Triangle Strategy? Fred Joyal over at Futuredontics, the parent company for 1-800-DENTIST, knows there is one such strategy. And it is this...

The phone should never be allowed to ring more than 3 times before it is answered....by a living, breathing human being.[28] When this strategy is made policy and incentive programs instituted to reward front desk team members for bringing in new patients, then magic starts happening for your practice. Imagine the confidence in your team patients will have when they know that when they call your office, the phone is always answered. The 3 Rings Rule is one of the major pillars that have contributed to Dr. Mark Costes' success as a multi-practice owner.

To take this to a whole new level, we know that people are online long after dental practices are closed. So, how about re-routing your calls to a call center during the hours and days when your office is closed? This will make sure that whether open or closed, somebody is always ready to answer the phone and when you factor the 3 Rings Rule, you add an extra dimension that makes patients know your team is on the ball.

We're living at a time when people expect to get things right when they want them and not be made to wait longer than is necessary. And when it comes to waiting for a phone call to get answered, anything over three rings is way too long. So make it a policy in your office to have the phone picked up in under three rings.

Fig 28: Dr. Money Bags vs Dr. Pickup Scraps

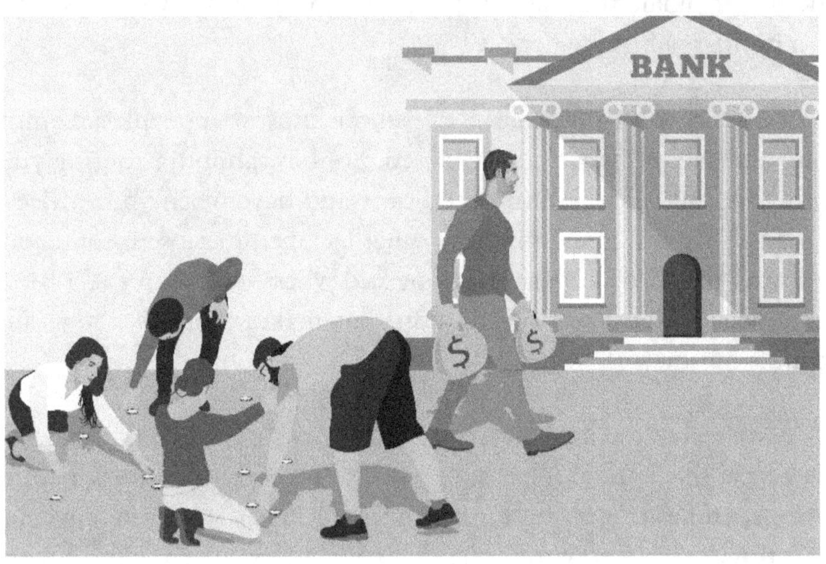

Having your Front Desk team make it a cardinal rule that the phone never rings three times before it's answered is the difference between the dentist holding two money bags on his way to the bank and the other four picking left-overs on the ground.

Do you want to be the dentist holding the money bags or be among the group gathering scraps on the ground? We have the money-bags-dentist plan. Reach out to us at www.9spe.com/contact. The choice is yours. One of the dentists in your area will be the one holding the money bags. I want it to be you.

ASK FOR PERMISSION FIRST

ALWAYS ASK FOR PERMISSION TO PUT YOUR CALLERS ON HOLD

When it comes to delivering a great customer service experience, it all comes down to the cumulative effect of every interaction that current and prospective patients have with members of your team at every touchpoint. Every detail therefore matters. As a Dentist who's bent on creating a patient experience that will put your practice in a class of its own, no detail is too small to ignore.

One such detail is how your staff puts callers on hold when a call comes in and the caller, unfortunately, has to be put on hold. What should never happen is for a caller to just be told, *"Thanks for calling XYZ Dental, please hold."* This is what should happen if your goal is to work till you're 95 years old.

If your goal, however, is to work less on the clinical side of your practice and retire early after selling your practice for multiple 7 figures, then the act of putting callers on hold has to be done with tact, always considering the caller's experience.

The first thing to do if a caller has to be put on hold is to ask for permission to put them on hold. Not that the caller has much of a choice, but the courtesy of seeking permission tells the caller two things. First, it tells them yours is a busy place and that's a good thing. Nobody wants to go into an empty restaurant when across the street there is one brimming with patrons. Second, it tells them you value their time, which makes them feel important.

When the caller has given the permission, you should give them a time frame for how long they will be on hold just in case they prefer you calling them back. Thank the caller for the permission and then proceed to put the call on hold. Handle what needs to be handled and return to the call in the time frame promised. Thank the caller, give them a sincere apology for making them wait and go right ahead to show them how excited and looking forward to their call you were.

There are many phone skills training programs out there. Find one that you and your team like and make the investment in your team's phone skills. This is easily the most critical choke point to your practice growth, so its mission critical that every aspect of phone interactions is world-class.

USE EXCITEMENT TO PULL THEM INTO YOUR OFFICE

HOW ANSWERING EVERY CALL LIKE YOU WERE LOOKING FORWARD TO IT MAKES CALLERS LOOK FORWARD TO COMING IN TO SEE YOU

I went for my Covid-19 test on a Friday. My appointment was at 3:30 pm. The test was held on the outskirts of Calgary a good 30 minutes' drive from my house. Even though there was no chance of traffic – thanks to the stay-at-home-orders – I left home early because I couldn't locate the address on Google maps. My anxiety level was also at an all-time high, so I wanted to remove any chances of me getting lost and missing the testing appointment.

I got there early and waited my turn to drive in. When my turn came, I drove in. After the less than 2 minutes testing process, I was told the results would be coming in five days or less. I would be getting one of two phone calls depending on the test result, the wonderful lady behind the glass face shield and mask informed me.

If I was positive, the call would be made by a live human being and if I was negative, I would get an automated call. I was told to be on the lookout for that call to make sure I would not miss it.

Given how important this call was to me and everyone else who got tested, there is no way on earth this call would be missed. I had already been living in isolation stuck in my daughter's room in the basement for three days, so there is no way I was going to miss that call.

Now given how much I was looking forward to this call, how many times do you think I allowed my phone to ring before I picked it up? My wife and kids were upstairs and even when their phones rang that Friday evening and Saturday morning, I called out asking if the call was mine. Just in case some wicked devil had taken hold of me and caused me to give the people at the testing center my wife or daughter's phone number instead of mine. Yeah, that's how much I was looking forward to the call.

The call came around 10 am the next day. I didn't even wait for the phone to ring. As soon as a number displayed, I clicked the answer button. As you can imagine, my life's direction going forward would depend on whether I was greeted with the normally hated – but today loved – tone of an automated message or the loved – but today hated – voice of a living human.

It was an automated message. "I DON'T HAVE CORONA YOU SUCKERS!" I shouted at the top of my lungs as I ran upstairs to hug my family.

Now, what does this story have to do with how phones are answered in your dental practice? A lot. Fred Joyal, the co-founder of 1-800-DENTIST, once said that 50% of prospects who call a dental office are lost on the first call they make. Why? Because the callers do not feel the person who answers them is genuinely excited and interested in them. The callers sense indifference in the voice and tone of the front desk team member who answers their calls and they make the decision to save themselves and their loved ones from that indifference by finding another dental office.

Horst Schulze, the co-founder of the Ritz-Carlton Hotel Company and the man responsible for its unrelenting pursuit of the 9-Star Experience, always maintained that customer service starts at the front door or with the first ring of the phone.[29] It's during those initial moments when a call is answered that the welcome-to-our-family experience gets, or fails to get demonstrated to the patient. The disposition of the team member who answers the phone must, with genuine sincerity, demonstrate to the caller how much she was looking forward to the caller's call.

During and after talking to people on the phone, anybody that makes a call into your office must feel beyond the shadow of any doubt that they called the right dental office. They must feel they belong there and must look forward to coming in, all because of how your front desk team demonstrated how much they were looking forward to the call that resulted in the appointment.

Fig 29: Excitement Must Show Through The Phone

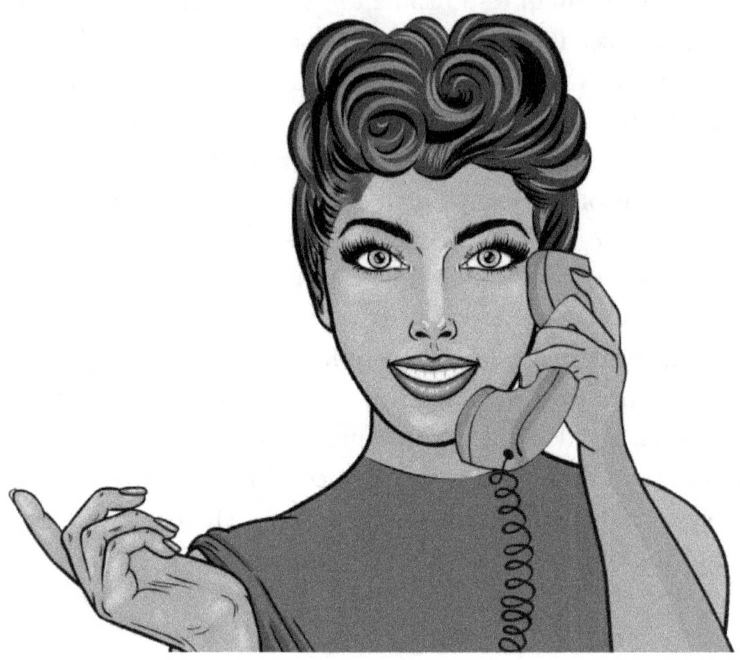

The smile and excitement of the person who answers the phone must show through to the person who made the call. The caller must feel the person who answers the phone was looking forward to their call.

WOW THEM WITH GENUINE INTEREST

WATCH OUT FOR KEYWORDS OVER THE PHONE AND WOW YOUR CALLERS WITH INTEREST

One of my favorite things to do is to call dental practices across North America to comparison test the level of customer service awareness demonstrated by their Front Desk teams. (My apologies to the hard-working front desk teams across North America that I have and will continue to put to the test)

One day I had the idea of testing to find out if any of the offices I called had their staff on the ball when it came to picking up on cues and keywords that would reveal that I am a potential new patient.

When I called, I'd introduce myself and let the person who picked up the phone know that my family and I just moved into the community and were looking for a dentist. To be sure, I said the exact same thing to everybody who answered the phone giving the following facts:

1. I was new to the city
2. I had moved with my family
3. We were looking for a dentist

What I was looking for was an office whose front desk would demonstrate the highest level of care and interest in me as a new member of the community. Of the 10 offices I called over two days, only one in downtown Toronto had the lady who answered the phone demonstrate the level of interest that would have turned my call into a booked consultation appointment. How did this lady achieve this over a short phone call?

She – in a voice that showed genuine interest – welcomed me and my family to the city. She then asked me where we had just moved from and the reason for our move. She then proceeded to ask if our kids were adjusting well. She had picked up the fact that we had kids because I had mentioned that my family and I had moved into the city.

After establishing great rapport and demonstrating a remarkably high level of interest in me, the lady asked me for the best day my family and I could come in to meet her "awesome dentist" (her exact words not mine) for our free consultation. I told her that I would discuss with my wife and get back to her.

If I was on a real search for a dentist, this office would most likely have deserved to be checked out in person. The lady did most of the right things right but she also did not do some critical things.

She never took down my email address or phone number. When I told her that I would discuss with my wife, she should have asked for my wife's number, so that she can follow up with her as well. She should have asked for my phone number as well as my wife's and obtained permission from me to send us a short text message just to confirm this conversation.

This is what 7 and 8-figure dental practices excel at. Their front desk staff has antennas that are always on the lookout, scanning for keywords that reveal great potential for new business. And when they get those cues, they deploy them to show genuine interest and care for the people they will be talking to.

How good is your team at picking up critical cues over the phone? Listen in to your calls and find out. If you're too swamped, get somebody else to listen in for you. It's the best way to train and help your front desk ninjas to become great at what they do.

DRIVE THE URGENCY TO HAVE TREATMENT DONE NOW

USE EVERYDAY LIFE ANALOGIES TO GIVE YOUR PATIENTS THE EXPERIENCE OF FULLY UNDERSTANDING THE LONG-TERM EFFECTS OF NOT STARTING TREATMENT RIGHT NOW

Most oral health issues that'll become chronic in the future, requiring large financial commitments to make them go away, take time to become chronic. By the time a person's teeth start falling out in their senior age, the problems will have been accumulating during the entire lifetime. But people don't understand this when it comes to their teeth. They understand this very well when it comes to things like their cars and homes.

Many dentists are reluctant to rub patients the wrong way by bringing up treatment options for problems that might be years away from becoming emergencies. When a patient comes for say, a regular cleaning and the assistant sees an alignment issue that might be solved by Invisalign, there is an understandable reluctance to bring this issue up for fear the patient might think you're just upselling them.

When asked by Dr. Paul Etchison how his team manages to present Invisalign to patients who would not have come in for Invisalign without sounding salesy – a not so great patient experience – Dr. Craig Spodak DDS, who runs Spodak Dental in Delray Beach, Florida, gave an excellent analogy. Every savvy dentist who wants to double or triple their case acceptance should swipe and deploy this analogy when presenting patients with treatment options.

According to Dr. Spodak, if you want to show patients the importance of taking a certain treatment now (without sounding salesy) if they want to keep their teeth after 20 years, bring the urgency of taking action now closer to home by giving them the analogy of getting an oil change for their vehicle.

Ask the patient if they normally wait for their car to stop running before they take it for oil change. Or if they wait for the roof on their house to collapse before fixing the small hole that a roofing inspector finds during the yearly roof checks. Most people will say no, they don't wait for their vehicles to break down before they take them in for an oil change. And most definitely, no homeowner will take a wait and see attitude to a hole on their roof. They'll get it fixed right away.

Demonstrating the importance of taking a certain course of action now using the verbiage of an analogy enables the patient to see the urgency of taking action now.

Fig 30: Crush Your Competition

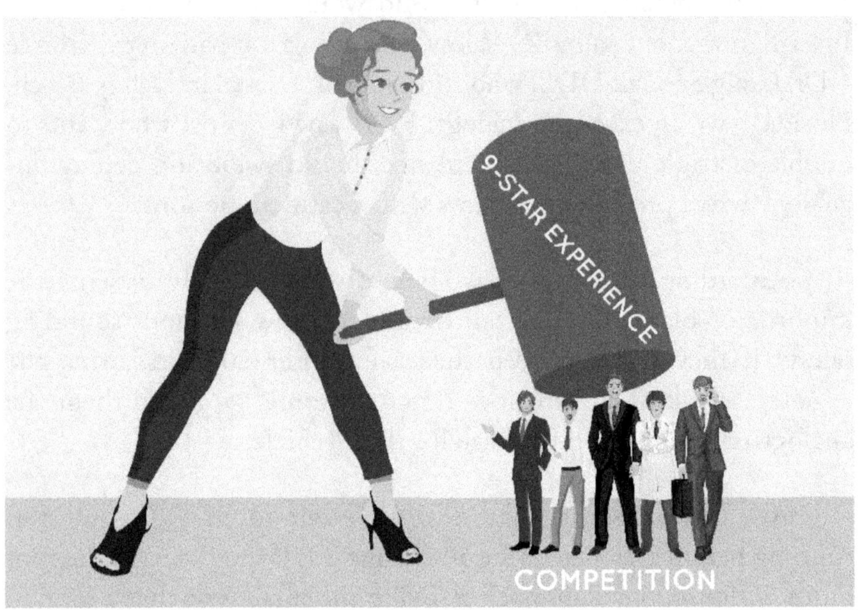

Delivering a world-class patient experience is like a huge hammer against the competition. And that competition is made up of not only other dentists. It's made up of anything that people spend money on that is not dentistry. When you give people more than commoditized dental services, you'll have become what Fred Joyal calls, a lifestyle enhancement service.[30] This is where you want to be. I can help you get there using The Dentistry Funnel Framework. **So, Doctor, who would you rather be? The one wielding the hammer or the one under the hammer?**

GIVE THEM ACCESS TO FINER THINGS

REDUCING PATIENTS' FEAR OF DENTISTRY BY GIVING THEM ACCESS TO UPSCALE SERVICES

Members of the human family have some of the weirdest beliefs when it comes to their oral health in general, and their teeth in particular. These beliefs are responsible for why fear is named as the main reason most people procrastinate or don't visit a dentist.

One of the smartest ways to dissolve this fear is to do what Dr. George K. Camp DDS, and Erika Wayne at Heritage Dental Spa & Salon in Bluffton, South Carolina, are doing.[31] Their dental patients have paid access to a high-end hair and nails salon as well as upscale spa treatment. When a dental appointment is packaged or offered with an optional spa or nails session, the resulting patient experience leads to amazing growth in referrals, new patient acquisition, consistently high recall rates and reduced patient churn.

Now, you might be thinking this is nice and good for the business savvy folks at Heritage Dental Spa & Salon because they already have these upscale assets as an integral part of their strategy. What about you, given that you don't have a spa, a hair or nail salon? How do you give your patients access to these services?

Simple. You create partnerships with providers of these services in your community. There is no business owner out there who will refuse the opportunity to partner with a busy dental office to refer clients. You will be surprised at how willing most of them are. Even to the extent of being able to offer your patients some great deals on such days as Valentine Week, Mother's Day, Father's Day, etc.

You can even go as far as creating an exclusive club made up of say, patients who received implants, veneers, or other treatments. You can be as creative as you want, all for the purposes of giving your patients an experience they will never get anywhere else. You could also make deals with these establishments so that you can give access to them as rewards for such business boosters as referrals or anniversary gifts.

GO VIRTUAL

MAKE IT SUPER CONVENIENT FOR PATIENTS TO GET CONSULTATIONS DONE BY HAVING A VIRTUAL CONSULTATION OPTION

Convenience is a particularly important driver of world-class patient experiences. That is why practices that have convenient hours will retire their owners earlier and with much bigger practice valuations than those who don't. One of the best ways to give your patients a very convenient way to have their consultations done is to deploy and offer a Virtual Consultation option.

At a time when social distancing has increased people's anxiety and fears of coming into public establishments like dental offices, the savvy dentist will thrive by offering patients the safe and convenient option of having their consultations done virtually.

There are many virtual dentistry options out there but one I've found to be most effective and easy to deploy in my view – you can check others on the market – is Smile Virtual. It is easy to set up, comes with an in-depth training master-class and allows everything to be done at the patient and the doctor's convenience.

By eliminating the need to come in and have the consultation done in the office, Virtual Consultations save patients time – a 9-Star Experience driver – while giving the flexibility to do the actual consult at your most convenient time.

ASK FOR PERMISSION FIRST

USE CONVENIENT HOURS TO DRIVE YOUR PATIENT EXPERIENCE TO A HIGHER LEVEL

One of the savviest moves deployed by the legendary Horst Schulze when he was going after delivering the most outrageous guest experience at the Ritz-Carlton Hotels was to give guests flexible check in and check out times. For travelling executives and families that didn't want to be rushed by the check-in and check-out deadlines, the ability to leave as and when they were ready proved to be, like I said, one of the savviest moves Mr. Schulze ever deployed.

As a dental practice, providing convenient hours is not just an act of marketing genius, it's a God-send gift for most parents. You know your practice, if you aren't already opening early and closing late on some days of the week and having some weekend days open, then this is some low hanging fruit you're passing up on. You will not achieve the flexibility and availability of a luxury hotel, but the experience and appreciation from your patients will be quite similar to that of the hotel guests.

SECTION 9

THE 9-STAR SOCIAL MEDIA EXPERIENCE

EXPLODE SAFETY AWARENESS

USE SOCIAL MEDIA TO MAKE PEOPLE FEEL SAFE TO COME IN TO SEE YOU AND YOUR TEAM

The strength of people's relationship with social media just increased a 1000X due to stay-at-home orders. Having been locked in doors for weeks, social media was the only link to the outside world and boy, did it deliver. Every social media platform witnessed an unprecedented spike in use and things are not returning to their pre-Covid days anytime soon. No sir!

While social media has enjoyed a meteoric rise in use, people's perception of safety in public places has taken a corresponding drop. So, what are you going to do to make people feel safe? Well, you'll do what most business savvy dentists are doing; you'll use social media to make people feel safe to come in.

You've obviously changed a lot of things in your practice to enhance safety according to the regulations that your governing body has laid out. Were you taking videos and pictures of the changes? If you have not, then please get started. You're already a wee bit late, but better late than never.

When you have the videos and pictures, post them on social media. Use them in your follow-up campaigns. Be seen going over and above the minimum requirements all in the name of your patients' safety and wellbeing. If people are going to be on social media more than ever before, then why not use social media to show them the lengths you and your team are going to ensure they are safe.

BE SUPER RESPONSIVE

RESPOND TO ALL SOCIAL MEDIA POSTS AND REVIEWS TO LET YOUR PATIENTS KNOW AND FEEL THEY ARE VALUED AND LISTENED TO.

Mary Kay Ash, the legendary direct sales cosmetics brand founder built her empire by making women feel great. She is famously quoted for having said that everyone walks around with a sign around their neck that says, make me feel important. I don't know about you, but it annoys me right off when I post a review or comment on a brand's Facebook or Google page and the people behind the brand never bother to acknowledge me.

When people are going through online reviews not only are they looking into what people say about you, your team, and your practice. They are also looking to see if you are grateful and decent enough to acknowledge those who take the time to engage with your brand in one way or another. Nobody likes to hang around ungrateful people and when your practice fails to acknowledge people's reviews and comments on social media, people consider that rude and ungrateful, exactly the kind of thinking you don't want people to have about you and your team.

It does sound petty I know, but people do want to be validated for things they get out their way to do. It makes us feel important, so you need to get your social media posts scanned for new posts and comments, so that those posts and comments are responded to. All this adds to creating a digital experience with your brand that both current and future patients relate and identify with as caring and attentive.

I was looking at Nelson Ridge Family Dental's Facebook and Google Review pages the other day. I was not impressed by the fact that every review post is responded to. This is how a great social media experience is deployed.

Fig 31: Respond To Social Media Reviews

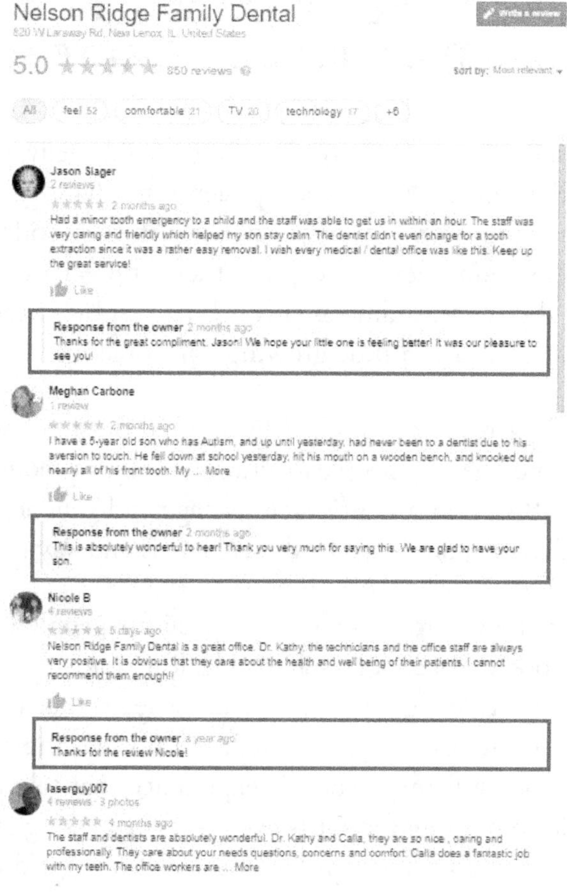

Moment of Magic #68

MAKE IT SUPER EASY TO LEAVE YOU REVIEWS

THE SECRET TO MAKING IT SUPER EASY FOR YOUR PATIENTS TO SAY GOOD THINGS ABOUT YOU...THE ONE CLICK STRATEGY

When you and your team have done a great job delivering a great dental experience, you want your patients to thank you not just by paying, staying with you, and referring their friends and loved ones. You also want them to express their appreciation by saying good things about you online as this is how you build the magnetic reputation needed to continue growing your practice.

If you do a really good job delivering an outstanding customer service experience, getting people to write good things about you online can be easier. But if your dentistry is average and generic, then you'll have an uphill battle, but it can be done. Here is one way to get it done.

The goal here is to make it super easy for people to leave you reviews on Google, Facebook, Yelp or Healthgrades. To succeed, you must make the review-giving experience so easy that even a grade three kid can do it. You know as much as I do that the modern-day adult human being is busy. So, any experience that takes her out of her way to do something for you – even if it's expressing gratitude for something that was to her own benefit – will not get done because it's a negative experience. That is why it's imperative for you to create a review generation process that does not need people to get out of their way to say good things about you online.

So how do you get this done? Easy. Just use the One Click Strategy for leaving reviews. With this strategy a review request message – text or email – is sent to the patient, and they have just to click one link that takes them straight to the Google or Facebook review page for your practice. The whole process to leave a review is so frictionless it could take 2-minute tops for a patient to leave a review.

Fig 32: Reviews Request Email

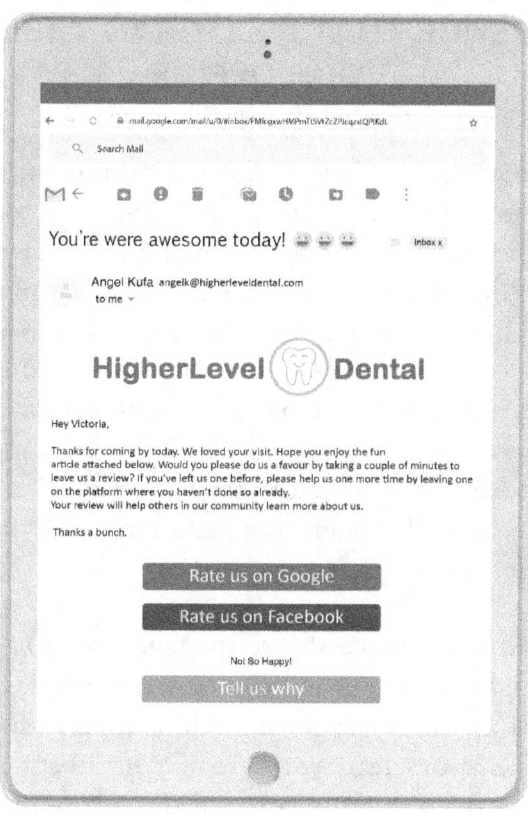

LEVERAGE THE POWER OF VIDEO

HOW TO DEPLOY THE AWESOME POWER OF VIDEO TO GIVE PATIENTS THE KIND OF DIGITAL EXPERIENCE THAT WILL DRAG THEM INTO YOUR OFFICE

The exponential rise in video content consumption - made even more exponential by the Coronavirus stay-at-home orders - presents a unique opportunity for the savvy dental practice owner to deliver one of a kind digital experience for current or future patients who come into contact with any of his or her online brand assets.

As always, it's all about being patient-centric. It's all about asking how best you can deploy the most effective assets that will give your patients an experience that will magnetically pull them into your office. A well-thought-out and strategically deployed video strategy will do this very well.

Many people are video-shy, so the reluctance to get in front of the camera might be an issue for a lot of dentists. To which I say this – get over it. To make it easy on yourself, partner with someone (we can help) to help you create your overall content strategy first, and then work with them to build your video asset library as part of an integrated authority building strategy.

Talk to your patients and staff and have them sign to agree to let you film them in compliance with HIPAA in the USA, PIPEDA in Canada, The Data Protection Act in the UK, GDPR in Europe or any privacy regulations where you operate. The last thing you want is to get yourself into a bowl of hot soup for violating privacy laws and regulations.

The first place to start when it comes to creating great video content is by creating videos of a welcoming and trust-building office tour. At a time when physical distancing presents challenges to doing physical office tours, a well-scripted digital tour of your office will do wonders in creating the kind of experience you want your patients to have.

The next sets of videos that you need to have created are Stories of Transformation videos. These are videos of patients talking about their challenges, fears, and pain before they had procedures done with you. These are powerful of case acceptance. The next set of videos are those of fun office activities, procedures, technology showcases as well as those highlighting any community events you do. Use every opportunity to create these video assets and then deploy them across your entire digital footprint.

LOVE ON YOUR PAID LEADS

PLEASANTLY SURPRISE PEOPLE THAT RESPOND TO YOUR FACEBOOK ADS

The number of dental practices using paid advertising as a new patient-acquisition strategy spiked exponentially as soon as the stay-at-home orders were loosened. As a savvy dental practice owner, or as one working hard towards becoming one, you know that for your paid advertising efforts to be considered effective, they have to result in people actually coming into your office to get the procedures you are advertising done.

Let's say that you are running ads for dental implants on Facebook. How can you create an experience that will ensure Nancy Woodworks, the 55-year-old social butterfly, actually shows up at your office after she has clicked on your ad and booked an appointment online? How do you - before you even meet her face to face - reach out and confirm to her that the decision to book an appointment after seeing your ad is one of the best decisions she has made?

See, the last thing Nancy expects after booking an appointment online is to get a voice mail and text message from the dentist congratulating her on the decision and welcoming her to the practice. I know of people that booked dental appointments after having seen ads on Facebook and never got anything from the advertisers. So, when Nancy gets your voice mail welcoming her to the family and reaffirming her wise decision, you bet she's going the think, "*Oh my, these people are awesome; I can't wait to meet them in person.*"

The chances of her cancelling or not showing up after you've pleasantly surprised her like this are incredibly low. Now, to buttress your efforts, you follow up this online booking and welcome messages by providing Nancy with great value in the form of a report titled, "*FINALLY EXPOSED…The secrets to using dental implants to shave 15 years off how you look & becoming the social magnet everyone wants to be like.*" Or, another one titled, *10 Reasons Why Smart Folk Like You Put Off Getting Implants & How That Decision Affects Their Mental Health and Drive Them To An Early Grave.*

You can be guaranteed that even if she doesn't read the entire report, she will be all over your website reading and watching the Stories of Transformation videos on your Implants Treatment Page. The automated welcome phone call, text message, and free reports that will be followed by a direct appointment confirmation from your team will seal the deal.

TURN UNHAPPY PATIENTS INTO RAVING FANS

CONVERTING AN UNHAPPY PATIENT WHO HAS LEFT A NEGATIVE REVIEW INTO A RAVING FAN OF YOUR PRACTICE

Negative reviews are a natural part of running a business. Most people dislike them because of the possible impact to one's reputation. But looked at with an eye towards delivering a 9-Star Experience, a negative review can be used to further solidify one's reputation.

There's one thing you MUST do to give an unhappy patient an experience that will convert them after they have voiced their unhappiness in the form of a negative review. Reach out to them as soon as the displeasure is voiced, or as soon as somebody on your teams discovers it. If the unhappy patient's social media profile has enough information to identify who they are (a lot of people use fake names on their social media profiles), then use whatever means is at your disposal to reach out to them. Find out from your team where exactly the delivery in service broke down and make moves to rectify the situation.

Like I said, the key is reaching out to the unhappy patient as quickly as possible. Avoid being defensive and do your absolute best to rectify the situation if it's possible to do so. Go over and beyond to show the patient what you've done to rectify the situation. This experience will, in most cases, result in the unhappy patient taking down the negative review and replacing it with a glowing testament of how you went to heaven and back to make things right with them.

For you and your team to be on top of the reviews that people are leaving on the various platforms, you'll need a good reviews management tool that will be able to give you a notification when a negative review has been left. That way, you'll be able to move with great speed to reach out to the patient and handle the situation.

Fig 33: Reviews Notification Text

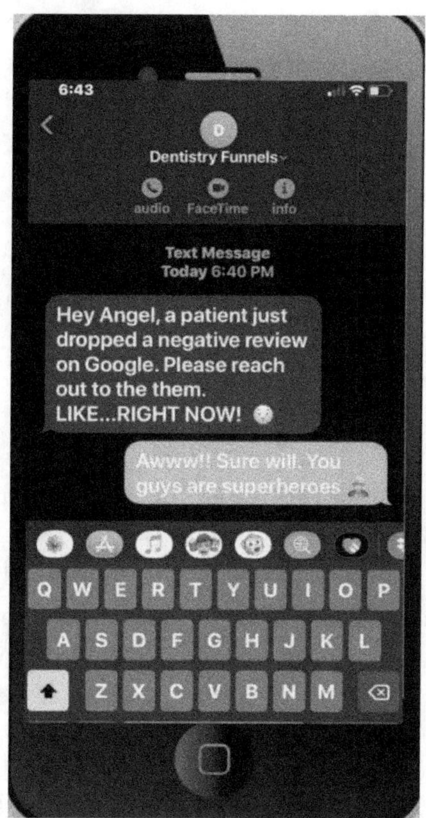

APOLOGIZE LIKE NO OTHER

WHEN THERE IS A BREAKDOWN IN SERVICE, APOLOGIZE LIKE NO OTHER

You're in a people-facing business, so I'm sure mistakes have happened. If none have happened yet, count yourself lucky but rest assured, mistakes will be made. What determines whether or not you get to keep a patient, or you don't get sued is what actions you take when a mistake has been made.

Whatever the severity of the mistake, it's important that you demonstrate that you care and are sorry for what happened. So, after you have done whatever is needed to redress the mistake, you want to go a step further and wow the patient using the following strategy.

Now, if you and your team had been doing a good job of recording all the pertinent information you can about your patients – favorite wine, flowers, champagne, books, food, etc. – then you would be in a really good position to know exactly what to use to sooth the pain that your mistake caused. If you don't know anything special that this wronged patient loves or likes, then that is alright as long as you execute on the Apologize Like No Other strategy.

Here is how you create an unforgettable Moment of Magic after you or a member of your team has fumbled the ball during Superbowl.

Buy two different high-quality apologies cards. One to be signed by every member of your team and one to be signed by just you as the Dentist. Next, buy a bottle or two of wine, champagne or a bouquet of flowers. Please don't go to your local grocery store for the flowers and don't you cheap out on the wine. The goal here is to show the patient that you care and are sorry for what happened.

Next, have every member of your team sign the apologies card and have a simple message on there. Something along these lines… *"Mrs. Smith, we just wanted to let you know how sorry we are for what happened yesterday. Please enjoy the wine."* As the dentist, you must write a heartfelt and sincere message on your card and sign it. When both cards are signed, get the wine bottle and flowers professionally packaged and have them couriered to Mrs. Smith's house.

Mrs. Smith will be more than pleasantly surprised to receive the gift. Receiving this gift over and above all the actions you and your team have taken to redress the mistake will go a long way in helping Mrs. Smith forgive you. Not only will you have drastically increased the odds that she will remain a loyal patient, you will have significantly lowered the number of people she will mention this mistake in a negative light to.

If a service provider makes a mistake and they go to these lengths to apologize how would you feel? Would you forgive them and give them a second chance? I would and so would most people.

CONCLUSION

I remember listening to a very instructional story of a successful dentist being interviewed on a podcast. I'm sorry, I don't remember which podcast or the name of the dentist, I listen to too many of these things. This dentist told the story of how he was struggling with the decision of whether or not to get into dental school. What got him into taking action – action that he is forever glad he took – is how his parents showed him how five years from the day they had the conversation was going to come by whether or not he took action.

Like dentist in this story, I'll be a good friend and tell you this. If you're struggling with the decision to take action on implementing the 9-Star Patient Experience strategies, know this. Three, five, or ten years from today will come. The important question to reflect upon is whether your practice will be better off with or without implementing some of the strategies that will, with 100% certainty, turn your patients into raving fans that pay more, refer a lot more, and stay with your practice their entire lifetime – or as long as they still live within driving distance of your practice.

As the world gets itself used to the new normal ushered in by the Coronavirus pandemic, two groups of dental practices will emerge. The first group will be made up of practices that struggle to get back to their pre-COVID production levels. The second group will be made up of practices that will not only get back to their pre-COVID production levels, but that will proceed to surpass them.

What will be the major differentiating factor between the two groups? Focus of a world-class patient experience. That's what the difference will be.

Having an uncompromising focus on giving your patients an experience like no other will be the main differentiator, because like it or not, a crown is a crown, braces are braces and teeth whitening is just what it is. Teeth whitening. Real differences in the actual deliverables that make up the practice of dentistry between one dentist and another are minimal. The main differentiator between your practice and everybody else's in your market is the experience that patients get. Ignore this truth and when the time comes, you will be looking to sell your practice for a fraction of what it could be worth had you taken heed of this truth and acted on it.

If on the other hand, you take heed of this truth and work to build your practice around delivering a 9-Star Experience, then chances are high that you will be retiring on a very very fat pay day and having impacted your community in ways that will change their lives forever.

ACKNOWLEDGEMENTS

No man or woman can, in truth, claim to be self-made. For somebody who crossed the oceans with nothing but a single suitcase of clothes and $200 in my pocket, I owe a lot to many people. I have not yet personally met most of the people whose guidance and mentorship I'm benefiting from because honestly, in this day and age, I don't believe that I need to meet somebody in person to benefit from their work and guidance.

I'm truly thankful first of all, to Debby Dale, the property manager at one of the buildings whose security and concierge services we looked after, for putting our company's name forward in the bidding for our first high-end property at 100 Yorkville. This opened the flood gates to many other high-end properties where we proved that delivering a very high level of customer service trumps every disadvantage a person has in business… including a thick African accent.

I want to thank Dan Kennedy for introducing me to the crazy world of Direct Response Marketing through his Magnetic Marketing System as well as his other works on copywriting. My view and understanding of why things sell changed drastically after our chance encounter on YouTube.

I'm eternally grateful to Dr. Dustin Burleson, Dr. David Moffet, Fred Joyal, Dr. Howard Farran, Dr. Rinesh Ganatra, Dr. Paul Etchison, Dr. Anissa Holmes, Dr. Justin Short, and many other dentistry heavy weights whose wealth of experience and knowledge continue to feed my still very hungry mind.

I also would like to thank Sabri Subi over at King Kong and Josh Nelson over at The Seven Figure Agency for teaching me how to build an agency the right way. Your genius gentleman has made all the difference for me. I owe you big time.

My current work with Dentistry Flywheels would not have been possible had it not been for Jim Collins and his breakthrough framework.

I would like to give a massive shoutout to Shaun Clark and the entire team at High Level. You guys are the bomb. Seriously. The platform you've created is going to make boat loads of money for my clients.

My eternal gratitude also goes to Parthiv Shah for his mentorship and guidance as well as giving me access to his very very deep reservoir of knowledge. My family and I will be forever indebted to you my friend.

Lastly and by no means least, I would like to thank whoever came up with the idea of the internet. Dude or girl… I'll give up my seat for you in heaven in case you don't make it there. Peace.

ABOUT THE AUTHOR

Farai Kufakwedu embodies the spirit of entrepreneurial first-generation immigrants who come to the first world. After migrating to Canada in 2001, he built his first business providing Ritz-Carlton type concierge services to upscale high-rise residential condos in Toronto. By focusing on providing white glove service experiences to his clients, the business grew to seven figures in three years.

Since exiting that business, Farai has been building brands online leveraging the Amazon third party seller platform. Farai's new company, dentistryflywheels.com helps dental practices grow by deploying momentum building direct response marketing strategies built around the dental practice flywheel.

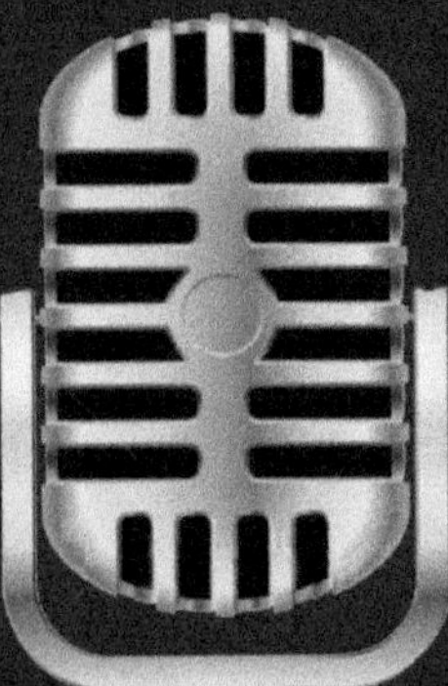

THE 9-STAR
PATIENT EXPERIENCE

Have You Liked
The Moments Of Magic
That You've Learned About
In This Book?

If So, Then Subscribe To My FREE Podcast
Called "The 9-Star Patient Experience"
Where Savvy Dentists Share Their Most
Effective Patient Experience Strategies.

You Can Subscribe For FREE
and get exclusive access to the most cutting
edge strategies and ideas at:

9spe.com/podcast

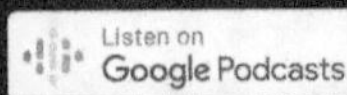

Listen on
Google Podcasts

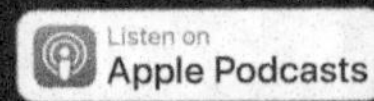

Listen on
Apple Podcasts

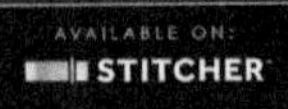

AVAILABLE ON:
STITCHER

Listen on
Spotify

ENDNOTES

SECTION ZERO

[1] Clason S, George. The Richest Man in Babylon. Berkley, 1988

[2] <u>Schulze</u>, Horst. Excellence Wins: A No-Nonsense Guide to Becoming the Best in a World of Compromise. Zondervan, 2019

[3] Moffet, David Dr. How To Add AT LEAST An Extra $100,000 In Billings To Your Dental Practice, Without Spending Even ONE Penny More... On Marketing, Extra Staff, Fancy Lasers, Or New Equipment!

[4] https://www.businesswire.com/.The Annual Customer Experience Impact (CEI) Report. January 11, 2012

[5] Short, Justin (Dr), Maloley, David (Dr). Titans of Dentistry: How the top performers think and act differently. Soapbox Publishing, 2018

[6] Maxwell, John C. The 21 Irrefutable Laws of Leadership: Follow Them and People Will Follow You. Thomas Nelson, 2007

SECTION ONE

[7] Joyal, Fred. Everything is Marketing: The Ultimate Strategy for Dental Practice Growth. Futuredontics Inc.2014

[8] Dorfman, Gina (DDS) "Elevate Your Patient Experience In Your Dental Practice" YAPI (Blog) Accessed May 2020

[9] Burleson, Dustin (DDS). The Ortho MBA Webinar. Watched May 22, 2020

[10] Moffet, David (Dr). How To Build The Dental Practice Of Your Dreams: (Without Killing Yourself!) Advantage Media Group, 2015

[11] Moffet, David Dr. How To Add AT LEAST An Extra $100,000 In Billings To Your Dental Practice, Without Spending Even ONE Penny More... On Marketing, Extra Staff, Fancy Lasers, Or New Equipment!

SECTION TWO

[12] Moffet, David (Dr). How To Build The Dental Practice Of Your Dreams: (Without Killing Yourself!) Advantage Media Group, 2015
[13] thousandoaksdentalspa.com/
[14] Moffet, David (Dr). How To Build The Dental Practice Of Your Dreams: (Without Killing Yourself!) Advantage Media Group, 2015

SECTION THREE

[15] Agarwal, Tarun (DDS), Place More Implants, Dental Heroes Podcast.

SECTION FIVE

[16] Takacs, Gary (DDS), Special Gift – Free Mouthguard Project Course for Thriving Dentist Show Listeners. Podcast Episode 436
[17] Witty, Adam and Shelton, Rusty. Authority Marketing: Your Blueprint to Build Thought Leadership That Grows Business, Attracts Opportunity, and Makes Competition Irrelevant. ForbesBooks, 2018
[18] Nelson Ridge Family Dental Facebook Page

SECTION SIX

[19] Burleson, Dustin (DDS). The Ortho MBA Webinar. Watched May 22, 2020

SECTION SEVEN

[20] Spodak, Craig (DDS). Becoming a Top Tier Invisalign Provider. Dental Heroes Podcast
[21] GKIC. Magnetic Marketing System

SECTION EIGHT

[22] Howard, Farran (DDS). Teamwork Makes The Dream Work With The Reflections Dental Care Team. Dentistry Uncensored Podcast. Watched April 2020
[23] Ganatra, Rinesh (DDS). Re-Inventing Dentistry: A new vision for building and marketing your dental practice. CreateSpace Independent Publishing Platform, 2013

[24] Joyal, Fred. Becoming Remarkable. Futuredontics, 2015

[25] Vo, Glenn (DDS). Running the Business VS. Building the Culture. Dental Heroes Podcast. Listened On 10 June 2020

SECTION NINE

[26] Makepeace, Clayton. Make Your Benefits Sparkle. Webinar. Watched January 2020

[27] Kennedy, Dan. Magnetic Marketing: How To Attract A Flood Of New Customers That Pay, Stay, and Refer. ForbesBooks, 2018

SECTION TEN

[28] Mark a. Costes, (DDS) Pillars of Dental Success: Systems and Strategies to Streamline the Marketing and Management of the Modern Dental Practice. Createspace, 2016

[29] Schulze, Horst. Excellence Wins: A No-Nonsense Guide to Becoming the Best in a World of Compromise. Zondervan, 2019

[30] Joyal, Fred. Everything is Marketing: The Ultimate Strategy for Dental Practice Growth. Futuredontics Inc.2014

[31] www.heritagedentalspa.com. Heritage Dental Spa & Salon. Page visited 12 May 2020